‹Rad Tech's Guide to

Equipment
Operation and
Maintenance

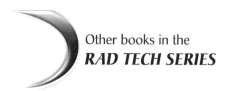

Other books in the
RAD TECH SERIES

Rad Tech's Guide to

Equipment Operation and Maintenance

Euclid Seeram, RTR, BSc, MSc, FCAMRT

Medical Imaging—Advanced Studies
British Columbia Institute of Technology
Burnaby, British Columbia
Canada

b

**Blackwell
Science**

© 2001 by Blackwell Science, Inc.

EDITORIAL OFFICES:
Commerce Place, 350 Main Street, Malden, Massachusetts 02148, USA
Osney Mead, Oxford OX2 0EL, England
25 John Street, London WC1N 2BL, England
23 Ainslie Place, Edinburgh EH3 6AJ, Scotland
54 University Street, Carlton, Victoria 3053, Australia

OTHER EDITORIAL OFFICES:
Blackwell Wissenschafts-Verlag GmbH, Kurfürstendamm 57, 10707 Berlin, Germany
Blackwell Science KK, MG Kodenmacho Building, 7-10 Kodenmacho Nihombashi,
    Chuo-ku, Tokyo 104, Japan
Iowa State University Press, A Blackwell Science Company, 2121 S. State Avenue,
    Ames, Iowa 50014-8300, USA

DISTRIBUTORS:
USA
  Blackwell Science, Inc.
  Commerce Place
  350 Main Street
  Malden, Massachusetts 02148
  Telephone orders: (800) 215-1000
      or (781) 388-8250;
  Fax orders: (781) 388-8270
Canada
  Login Brothers Book Company
  324 Saulteaux Crescent
  Winnipeg, Manitoba R3J 3T2
  Telephone orders: (204) 837-2987

Australia
  Blackwell Science Pty, Ltd.
  54 University Street
  Carlton, Victoria 3053
  Telephone orders: 03-9347-0300
  Fax orders: 03-9349-3016
Outside North America and Australia
  Blackwell Science, Ltd.
  c/o Marston Book Services, Ltd.
  P.O. Box 269
  Abingdon
  Oxon OX14 4YN
  England
  Telephone orders: 44-01235-465500
  Fax orders: 44-01235-465555

Acquisitions: Beverly Copland
Development: Julia Casson
Production: GraphCom Corporation
Manufacturing: Lisa Flanagan
Marketing Manager: Toni Fournier
Cover and interior design: Dana Peick, GraphCom Corporation
Typesetting: GraphCom Corporation
Printed and bound by Western Press

Printed in the United States of America
01 02 03 04 5 4 3 2 1

The Blackwell Science logo is a trade mark of Blackwell Science Ltd., registered
at the United Kingdom Trade Marks Registry.

        Library of Congress Cataloging-in-Publication Data

Seeram, Euclid.
    Rad tech's guide to equipment operation and maintenance / by Euclid Seeram.
      p. ; cm.
    Includes bibliographical references (p.   ).
    ISBN 0-86542-482-9
    1. Radiography, Medical—Equipment and supplies.
    [DNLM: 1. Radiography—instrumentation. 2. Quality Control. WN 150 S453r
  2001] I. Title: Guide to equipment operation and maintenance. II. Title.
  RC78.5 .S437 2001
  616.07'572—dc21

                                                          00-067464

This book is dedicated with love and affection to all my smart and wonderful nieces and nephews, listed in alphabetical order.

Adam McGreggor
Anne Penner
Cameron Liddell-Grainger—my great nephew
Christian Iversen
Dana Penner
Garry "Chip" Teekah
Hannah McGreggor
Helen Liddell-Grainger
Holly Febbraro
Jennifer Febbraro
Jessica Penner
Meghan Penner
Natalia Teekah
Nicholas Iversen
Ruth Bright
Sarah Febbraro
Stacie Seeram
Tasha Seeram
Trish Penner
Wendy Penner

TABLE OF CONTENTS

PREFACE

Equipment and quality control are essential core subjects of radiologic technology programs. To meet the needs of these programs, a handful of books on radiographic equipment and quality control are currently available to enable students and technologists alike to acquire the skills required to produce diagnostic quality images using radiation exposures as low as reasonably achievable.

In the changing health care environment and, in particular, in the evolution and development of varying degrees of occupational restructuring, there is a need to maintain and enhance technologist competency in a wide variety of areas. *Rad Tech's Guide to Equipment Operation and Maintenance* addresses this need by providing a comprehensive practical guide for technologists engaged in the art and science of equipment operation and quality control. An equally important consideration is the need for a single volume that provides students in training with a brief, clear, and concise coverage of the subject in preparation for their professional certification examination.

Rad Tech's Guide to Equipment Operation and Maintenance is not a textbook, and it is not intended to replace the vast resources on radiographic instrumentation and quality control. Rather, it provides a precis of the extensive coverage of essential core topics for technologists.

Rad Tech's Guide to Equipment Operation and Maintenance contains 10 short chapters that cover a wide scope of topics on equipment operation and quality control. Chapter 1 deals with the nature and scope of imaging systems for diagnostic radiology and sets the framework for the rest of the chapters. Whereas Chapter 2 presents a description of radiographic imaging systems, Chapter 3 describes the design and function of x-ray generators in detail. Chapter 4 outlines the characteristics of x-ray tubes and how they work. Chapters 5 and 6 address x-ray beam filtration and the principles of x-ray exposure timers, respectively. Additionally, Chapter 7 provides a description of antiscatter devices. Fluoroscopic imaging principles and instrumentation are discussed in Chapter 8. Chapter 9 reviews the types of mobile imaging systems and the principles of operation. Finally, Chapter 10 outlines the basic principles of quality control for radiographic imaging systems and focuses on tolerance limits for various quality control tests.

Enjoy the pages that follow and remember—your patients will benefit from your wisdom.

Euclid Seeram, RTR, BSc, MSc, FCAMRT
British Columbia, Canada

ACKNOWLEDGMENTS

Writing a technologist guide such as this one demands a great deal of understanding of the wide and varied resources currently available in the literature, as well as a perception of the contributions of the experts in the fields of radiographic instrumentation and quality control.

First, I must acknowledge Chris Davis, Executive Editor, who worked at Blackwell Science and who conceived the *Rad Tech Series* idea. Thanks, Chris, for selecting me as "the man for this project" and for all your warm support throughout the years. In addition, Julia Casson, Developmental Editor at Blackwell Science, kept me on track throughout the project. Thanks, Julia. I appreciate your efforts.

I am indeed grateful to all those who have dedicated their energies in providing several comprehensive volumes on imaging equipment and quality control issues for the radiologic community. First, I would like to acknowledge the notable medical physicist, Dr. Stewart Bushong, a professor of Radiologic Science in the Department of Radiology, Baylor College of Medicine, Houston, Texas, from whom I have learned a great deal on radiologic science. In addition, I have gained further insight into the nature, scope, and depth of quality control from Joel Gray, PhD, a medical physicist in the Department of Radiology, Mayo Clinic and Foundation, Rochester, Minnesota, through his written works on this topic.

To all others, such as the authors whose papers I have cited and referenced in this book, and to all the x-ray equipment manufacturers, thank you for your significant contributions to the knowledge base of these two important subjects. Additionally, I would like to express my sincere thanks to the publishers of these resources for their permission to reproduce relevant materials from their copyrighted works.

I am also grateful to Dana Peick and her production team at GraphCom Corporation. Thanks for your excellent work.

Finally, I must acknowledge the warm and wonderful support of my family, my lovely wife, Trish, a very caring person, and my smart and handsome son, David, a very special young man; thanks for your love. You both are indeed two of my life's treasures.

Last, but not least, I want to express my gratitude to all the students in my equipment and quality control classes—your questions have provided me with a further insight into teaching these important subjects.

—ES

CHAPTER 1

X-Ray Imaging Systems for Diagnostic Radiology

Chapter at a glance

The discovery of x-rays in 1895 by W.C. Roentgen led to the subsequent development of diagnostic radiology: the use of x-rays to produce images of the human body. These images are then interpreted by a radiologist who provides a diagnosis of the patient's medical condition.

Currently, there are a large number of systems to provide images of the human body using x-rays, ranging from systems that use simple film-screen technology to systems that use computer-based technologies.

This chapter first provides an overview of x-ray imaging systems, followed by an identification of the major components of radiographic, fluoroscopic, and mobile x-ray systems. These components are examined in greater detail in the other chapters of this book. Additionally, total quality management tools and techniques that ensure optimal performance of x-ray imaging systems are highlighted.

It is important that the technologist has a firm understanding of these major components and how they are integrated to provide diagnostic quality images.

IMAGING SYSTEMS OVERVIEW

Imaging systems for use in diagnostic radiology include radiography, fluoroscopy, conventional tomography, mobile radiography and fluoroscopy, mammography, and digital imaging systems.

Radiography

In *radiography*, x-rays pass through the body and strike an image receptor to produce a latent image that is rendered visible when the film is processed using chemical solutions.

- The source of x-rays is an x-ray tube.
- The x-ray beam from the x-ray tube passes through the body. Part of this beam is absorbed or attenuated by the body, and the remainder is transmitted through the body to strike the image receptor.
- The image receptor is a film-screen system that converts the transmitted x-rays to light photons. These light photons produce the latent image on the film.
- The latent image is rendered visible by chemical processing.
- Attenuation of the x-ray beam as it passes through the body is responsible for the formation of the image on the film. When a structure absorbs more x-rays, it will appear white on the film (after processing), compared with a structure that absorbs little x-rays (and allows more transmission of the beam). More x-rays falling on the film will produce more film blackening after processing.

■ The characteristics of the image that make it diagnostic are the contrast, detail, and noise. These characteristics not only depend on the performance of the imaging system, but also on the knowledge and skills of the technologist.

To date, radiography is the most common imaging system used to produce images in the radiology department.

Fluoroscopy

A *fluoroscopic imaging system* allows the radiologist to observe and study the dynamics or motion of organ systems. This process is possible because the system allows for direct observation of the human body on a television monitor. The images produced during fluoroscopy are continuous images as opposed to static images produced in radiography.

■ The source of x-rays in fluoroscopy is an x-ray tube.

■ The x-ray tube is energized for longer periods in fluoroscopy allowing for continuous production of x-rays during the examination.

■ The image receptor in fluoroscopy is the image intensifier tube, a highly specialized tube that converts x-rays to light.

■ The light is captured by a television camera tube or charge-coupled device (CCD) and converted to an electrical signal (voltage).

■ This signal is sent to a television monitor that converts the signal into a television image.

■ The image viewed on the television monitor can be recorded on film using a technique called spot filming.

■ Spot filming can be accomplished using a cassette-loaded spot film or a photo-spot camera.

Digital fluoroscopy (DF) is another common imaging system used in diagnostic radiology. This system is outlined in detail in Chapter 7.

Conventional Tomography

Tomography is a technique whereby the x-ray tube and image receptor move at the same time and in opposite directions. The purpose of this movement is to defocus structures above and below the layer of interest (focal plane). This layer of interest is the thickness of tissue known as the tomographic layer.

Conventional tomography is becoming obsolete with the introduction of computed tomography. However, linear tomography, as opposed to multi-directional tomography, is still being used in some hospitals.

The following points are important and play a role in optimizing the tomographic examination:

- The fulcrum is the point at which the x-ray tube and image receptor pivot during the examination.
- The tomographic layer, or layer of interest, is the object plane. The fulcrum is always located in the object plane.
- The thickness of the tomographic layer is defined by the tomographic angle. As this angle increases, the section thickness decreases.
- Thicker sections are imaged using angles that range from 0 to 10 degrees. In this case, the technique is referred to as zonography.

The overall goal of conventional tomography is to improve image contrast by blurring objects above and below the layer of interest thus enhancing subject contrast.

Mobile X-Ray Imaging

Mobile x-ray imaging includes systems developed by both radiography and fluoroscopy. These units are also referred to as portable x-ray units.

- The purpose of these units it to meet the needs of patients who are confined to their hospital beds as a result of severe trauma, pathology, or other related medical problems.
- Portable x-ray machines are mounted on wheels enabling the technologist to easily transport them to the patient's bedside.
- The main components of radiographic and fluoroscopic portable units are identified in the next section of this chapter.
- When operating portable x-ray machines, there are a number of important practical considerations that must be observed. These relate not only to the technical aspects of machine operation, but also to image quality parameters and radiation protection of patients and personnel. These considerations are described in detail in Chapter 9.

Mammography

Mammography is an example of soft tissue radiography. Specifically, mammography is radiography of the breast. There are specific technical requirements for mammography, including:

- **X-ray spectrum.** This spectrum is different from the spectrum used in conventional radiography. The useful beam of x-rays emitted by a mammographic x-ray tube must be capable of maximizing differential absorption of the soft tissues of the breast to optimize image contrast.

- **Range.** The range of the kilovolts (kV) used in mammography is between 20 kVp and 36 kVp in 1 kVp increments.

- **Tube.** A mammographic x-ray tube is a special tube using a molybdenum or rhodium target.

- **Quality.** Filtration of the beam is an important way to produce good quality images of the breast. For this reason, various target-filter combinations are used, such as molybdenum-molybdenum, molybdenum-rhodium, and rhodium-rhodium.

- **Image contrast.** The use of a grid in mammography is essential to enhance image contrast. Low ratio grids of 4:1 and 5:1 are typical.

- **Compression device.** This is an essential component of a mammographic system. The purpose of compression is to improve image quality and reduce the radiation dose to the patient.

- **Image receptor.** The use of the appropriate image receptor contributes to the image quality during the examination. Film-screen technology, particularly single-emulsion film, improves both image contrast and detail.

Mammography is not described further in this book; it is covered in a separate text in the "Rad Tech Series" of books.

Digital Imaging

Digital imaging is a term used to describe systems that use computers to process the data obtained from a patient. Digital imaging refers to imaging without film and overcomes the limitations of film-based systems.

Digital imaging systems include each of the following:

- Digital fluoroscopy (DF)

■ Digital radiography (DR)
■ Computed tomography (CT)
■ Magnetic resonance imaging (MRI)
■ Picture archiving and communication systems (PACS)
■ Teleradiology

Digital imaging systems are not described further in this book (with the exception of digital fluoroscopy); they are discussed in a separate text in the "Rad Tech Series" of books.

MAIN COMPONENTS OF AN IMAGING SYSTEM

An x-ray imaging system, whether for radiography, fluoroscopy, or mobile imaging, consists of several components systematically arranged to optimize performance during a radiologic examination. Each component plays a significant role in the production of the image. To optimize image quality and minimize radiation dose to patients and personnel, it is mandatory that technologists have a firm understanding of the purpose of each of the components and how they work together.

A typical x-ray imaging system is illustrated in Figure 1-1 and consists of the following major components:

■ *X-ray source.* This component refers to the x-ray tube, an integral part of the system and an important tool for the technologist. The purpose of the tube is to provide an appropriate beam of x-rays suited to the requirements of the particular examination.

■ *Imaging object.* There are two types of objects: the patient and test phantoms. As the x-rays pass through the objects, it is attenuated and scattered. The resulting transmitted x-rays contain information about the internal structures of the object and serve as the basis for image formation. Test phantoms are used to measure equipment performance and are an integral element to a quality assurance program.

■ *Image receptor system.* The image receptor refers to the detection system, the purpose of which is to detect or capture the transmitted x-rays from the patient or test phantom. Once the x-rays are captured, the x-ray photons are converted into a visible image. In film-based radiography, the image receptor is the screen-film cas-

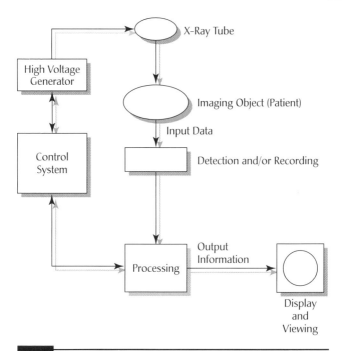

Figure 1-1 The essential components of an x-ray imaging system.

sette, and, in filmless imaging systems, is a digital detector. In fluoroscopy, the image receptor is the image intensifier tube, which detects transmitted x-rays from the patient and converts them into a high-intensity image.

- *Image processing system.* The data detected by the image receptor are not useful and must be processed to render the information visible for viewing by an observer. There are two types of processing systems: a chemical processing system and a computer processing system. The former contains chemical solutions for developing, fixing, and washing the film; the computer processing system is a digital computer that uses special computer programs (algorithms) to process the data it receives from the detector system.

- *Display and viewing system.* Once data are processed to generate images, the images must be displayed for viewing and interpretation. Two types of display devices are in use today: view boxes (also referred to as illuminators) and computer monitors. Although view boxes facilitate image display and viewing using a high-intensity light (from fluorescent tubes), their brightness levels cannot be changed. The observer cannot change the image brightness or contrast. Computer monitors are the display devices in a digital radiology department. These monitors are part of a computer workstation that features a powerful computer to allow observers to manipulate the image (using various algorithms) to suit their viewing requirements for the purpose of enhancing diagnostic interpretation.
- *High-voltage generator.* The purpose of this generator is to provide the high voltage to the x-ray tube to produce x-rays. Various types of generators are available, each offering its own unique set of advantages and disadvantages.
- *Control unit.* This unit is often referred to as the control panel. The purpose of the control panel is to allow the operator (technologist) to select and control various parameters that affect both the image quality and the radiation dose to the patient. For example, the technologist must select the exposure factors, kVp, milliamperage (mA), and time that are appropriate to the requirements of the examination. The control panel is vital to the imaging system because it provides visual evidence that appropriate factors have been selected and that the machine (the imaging system) is in proper working condition.

Each of these components are described further in later chapters, excluding film-screen image receptors.

It is important to note that the purpose of the imaging system is to produce optimal image quality and is under the direct control of the operator. Poor image quality, however, can occur and be attributed to operator error, uncooperative patients, and system performance problems.

To prevent and minimize system performance problems, equipment maintenance is necessary and is the mandate of a total quality management program.

QUALITY MANAGEMENT: AN OVERVIEW

Total quality management is an integral part of the daily activities in radiology and is considered a component of a continuous quality improvement (CQI) program. The notion of CQI
was developed by the Joint Commission on the Accreditation of
Healthcare Organizations (JCAHO) in 1991. CQI ensures that
every employee plays a role in ensuring a quality product.
Other terms synonymous with CQI are:

- Total quality management (TQM)
- Total quality improvement (TQI)
- Total quality control (TQC)
- Total quality leadership (TQL)

Before the introduction of the concept of CQI, other systems
were in place to ensure quality patient care in hospitals. In
radiology in particular, quality assurance and quality control
programs are essential, not only for optimizing the assessment
and evaluation of patient care, but also for monitoring the performance of equipment.

Quality Assurance

Quality assurance (QA) is a term used to describe systems and
procedures for ensuring quality patient care. QA deals specifically with quality assessment, continuing education, the use-
fulness of quality control procedures, and the assessment of
outcomes. QA deals with the administrative aspects of patient
care and quality outcomes.

Quality Control

Quality control (QC) is a component of QA and refers specifically to the monitoring of important variables that affect
image quality and radiation dose. QC involves the technical
aspects (rather than the administrative aspects) of equipment
performance.

Purpose of a CQI Program

The purpose of the procedures and techniques of CQI, QA, and
QC is threefold:

- To ensure optimal image quality for the purpose of
  enhancing diagnosis

- To reduce the radiation dose to both patients and personnel
- To reduce costs to the institution

NATURE OF QUALITY CONTROL

QC involves a number of activities that are significant to the technologist, particularly if the technologist is in charge of the QC program. These activities include acceptance testing, routine performance, and error correction.

- *Acceptance testing.* This is the first major step in a QC program, ensuring that the equipment meets the specifications set by the manufacturers.
- *Routine performance.* This step involves performing the actual QC test on the equipment with varying degrees of frequency (annually, semiannually, monthly, weekly, or daily).
- *Error correction.* This step ensures that equipment that does not meet the performance criteria or tolerance limit established for specific QC tests be replaced or repaired to meet tolerance limits.

Parameters for QC Monitoring

QC programs have been well established for radiography, fluoroscopy, film processing, and other imaging modalities such as computed tomography, mammography, nuclear medicine, ultrasound, and magnetic resonance imaging.

It is not within the scope of this chapter to describe the elements of these QC programs. However, a few important points are highlighted.

Parameters for radiographic QC testing include filtration, collimation, focal spot size, kVp accuracy, mA linearity, exposure timer accuracy, exposure reproducibility, screen-film contact, lead apron integrity, and the brightness level of view boxes and accessory equipment.

Fluoroscopy QC includes an assessment of exposure rate, spot-film exposures, and automatic exposure systems. In particular, fluoroscopic QC should begin with visual inspection of the components in the imaging chain and performance testing.

Visual inspection should include a checklist of several items, such as:

- Protective curtain
- Bucky slot cover
- Exposure switch and fluoroscopic timer
- Compression device
- Collimation shutters
- Table angulation
- Lead aprons and gloves

Performance testing should include:

- Reproducibility of exposure
- Focal spot size
- kVp accuracy and mA linearity
- Maximum exposure rate
- High- and low-contrast resolution
- Spatial resolution
- Image noise

Last, but not least, is processor quality control. This QC program is essential to ensure high-quality images and includes:

- Processor cleaning of racks on a daily and weekly basis.
- Processor maintenance to include both scheduled and preventive operations to ensure processor integrity.
- Processor monitoring of temperatures and replenishment rates of the various solutions, such as the developer and fixer. Equally important are sensitometry and densitometry measurements to address variables such as film contrast, density, speed, and base plus fog.

Quality Control Test Tools

There are numerous test tools currently available for QC programs in radiology. Examples of these tools include:

- *Sensitometer*. This instrument exposes a test filmstrip to a reliable, uniform, and reproducible light exposure for the purpose of processor monitoring.
- *Densitometer.* This instrument measures the density values of the sensitometer strip.
- *Penetrometer or step wedge.* This aluminum step-wedge can be used to check numerous variables.

- **Collimator test tool.** This tool is used to check the accuracy of the collimator.
- **Digital dosimeter.** This ionization chamber dosimeter is used to check a range of variables, including kVp accuracy, mA and time linearity, and mA and time in seconds (mAs) reciprocity.
- **Resolution test patterns.** These patterns measure the focal spot sizes of the x-ray tube.
- **Wire-mesh test pattern.** This pattern tests film-screen contact.

Control Charts

Control charts are important in a QC program. They provide graphic illustrations of a particular variable plotted as a function of time. Control charts provide a means of analyzing data that can generate information on trends. These charts can also demonstrate whether values meet or exceed upper and lower control limits. Corrective action must be taken when these limits fall outside a ± value.

Tolerance Limits or Acceptance Criteria

When a QC test is performed, the results should reflect proper operating levels when the imaging system is performing properly. An operating level is the level selected by the operator for the particular examination (e.g., 70 kVp). The tolerance limits or acceptance criteria are established objectively and subjectively and are values that define an upper limit of performance (a + value) and a lower limit of performance (a − value) that is acceptable. If the results fall outside this ± value, then the equipment fails the acceptance criteria test and must be repaired or replaced. For example, if a technologist conducts a QC test for kVp and the operating kVp selected was 70, then the results of the test would be acceptable only if the values fall within ± 4 kVp (Bushong, 2001). Therefore one would accept the QC test when the result is 74 or 66 kVp.

Other Considerations

Quality control programs must also take into consideration:

- **Record keeping.** Record keeping maintains the overall quality of the program.

- *Education and resources.* These sources must be made available to staff members so that they (the staff) may contribute effectively to the program.
- *Policy and procedure manual.* This manual ensures program coherence and defines the protocols of the QA-QC-CQI program.

CHAPTER 2

Radiographic Imaging Systems

Chapter at a glance

Radiographic imaging systems refer to x-ray machines installed in the main radiology department in the hospital. Technologists use these machines on a daily basis to produce diagnostic images of patients undergoing a wide range of routine x-ray examinations.

The purpose of this chapter is to present a description of the major components of a radiographic imaging system that play a role in the production of radiographic images. In addition, the main steps of film processing are highlighted and four factors influencing image quality are reviewed.

An understanding of these topics provide the technologist with the basic tools necessary to:

- Produce optimal image quality.
- Keep the radiation dose to the patient as low as reasonably achievable.
- Assess radiographic image quality.

MAJOR COMPONENTS OF A RADIOGRAPHIC IMAGING SYSTEM

The major components of a radiographic imaging system include an x-ray generator, an x-ray tube, a filter, a beam-limiting device, the x-ray beam itself, the patient, an x-ray table, a grid, an image receptor, and a film processing system (Figure 2-1). Additionally, the operator, or technologist, is an integral part of the imaging process. The technologist plays a central role not only in the care of the patient, but also in optimizing the use of the system to ensure the best possible image quality with the least amount of radiation dose. The interface between the electronics of the imaging system and the patient is the operator control console.

X-Ray Generator
A major part of the imaging system electronics is the x-ray generator.

- The purpose of the generator is to deliver electrical power to the x-ray tube to produce an x-ray beam suited to the goal of the examination. For example, if the x-ray examination, such as a chest, requires a short exposure time, then the generator allows the technologist to select and use this technique setting.
- The x-ray generator consists of several electrical components to change the electrical power from the utility company into a form suitable for x-ray production and control. Two of these components are transformers and rectifiers.
  - ❏ Transformers can be step-up or step-down devices. A step-up transformer increases the low voltage from

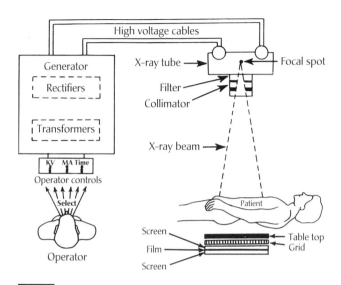

Figure 2-1 The major components of a radiographic imaging system. *(Reproduced with permission from Sprawls P. Principles of radiography for technologists. Gaithersburg, MD: Aspen Publishers, 1990.)*

the utility company (120, 240, or 440 volts) to high voltage (25 kilovolts to 150 kilovolts), which is required for x-ray production. A step-down transformer decreases the current and voltage from the utility company to levels suitable for energizing the x-ray tube.

❏ Rectifiers are electrical devices in the generator circuit that change the alternating current (AC) from the utility company into a direct current (DC) through a process referred to as rectification. Rectification allows electrons in the x-ray tube to flow in only one direction, that is, from cathode to anode. This is an important requirement for x-ray production.

The x-ray generator also allows the technologist to select and control the exposure technique required for the examination from the control console. The exposure technique determines the quality and quantity of the x-ray beam emanating from the x-ray tube.

These exposure technique factors include kilovoltage (kV), milliamperage (mA), and exposure time.

- kV controls the penetrating power of the photons in the x-ray beam. This penetrating power or beam quality is dependent on the size of the patient and the type of examination. Larger patients will require higher kV techniques to penetrate them and onto the film. The kV is the major controlling factor for image contrast.
- mA is the flow of electrons from cathode to anode. The mA controls the quantity of photons in the x-ray beam and influences the density of the image (or degree of film blackening).
- Exposure time (in seconds) is the duration of the x-ray exposure, which also determines the film density.
- The product of the mA and time in seconds (mAs) affects film density.

The x-ray generator allows the technologist to select the type of focal spot to be used for the particular examination. This aspect is important since the focal spot affects the sharpness of the image (image detail) and the amount of electrical loading (kilovolts peak [kVp] and mA and time in seconds [mAs]) that can be applied to the tube.

There are four basic types of generators: single-phase, three-phase, high-frequency, and constant potential generators. These are described in greater detail in Chapter 3.

X-Ray Tube

The x-ray tube is one of the most significant components in the imaging system and is an essential tool for radiographic and fluoroscopic imaging. The technologist therefore must have a firm understanding of what the tool is and how it works.

The x-ray tube uses the power from the generator to produce the x-ray beam required for the examination. There are two types of x-ray tubes, the basis of which depends on the anode design:

- Stationary anode tubes
- Rotating anode tubes

An x-ray tube (stationary or rotating) consists of the following components:

- *Anode.* This component is the positive electrode of the tube, which includes a target or focal spot that produces the x-ray beam when struck by electrons.

- ■ *Cathode.* This component is the negative electrode of the tube, which consists of a tungsten filament (wire) which, when heated, emits electrons. These electrons are subsequently accelerated at high speeds across the tube to strike the focal spot.
- ■ *X-ray tube insert.* The insert can be made of glass (glass envelope) or metal (metal envelope) and is designed to house or hold in place both the anode and the cathode structures.
- ■ *X-ray tube housing.* The housing is a metal cylinder in which the insert is placed. The housing serves a number of functions, including providing mechanical support for the insert.

The x-ray tube is described in detail in Chapter 4.

X-Ray Filters

A filter is a thin, flat piece of metal (e.g., aluminum) placed outside the x-ray tube. The purpose of a filter is to protect the patient by removing low-energy x-ray photons from the x-ray beam. These photons are absorbed by the patient because they do not have enough penetrating power to pass through the patient and onto the film. This removal of photons from the beam is known as filtration. There are three types of filtration: inherent, added, and total.

- ■ *Inherent filtration* is filtration from the glass envelope (insert), oil, and the window of the tube housing. This type of filtration is fixed; the technologist has no control of the amount of inherent filtration.
- ■ *Added filtration* can be added to the beam by the technologist. Certain examinations require a certain thickness of filter.
- ■ *Total filtration* is the sum of the inherent and added filtration. In general, the minimum total filtration for most radiographic examinations is 2.5 mm aluminum equivalent.

Beam-Limiting Devices

A beam-limiting device is used in imaging systems to determine the size and shape of the x-ray beam. This device is attached to the x-ray tube.

- ■ The purpose of beam limitation is to protect the patient by restricting the beam to the area of interest, or field-

of-view (FOV), as it is sometimes identified. There are
several types of beam-limiting devices, including cones,
cylinders, diaphragms, and collimators. Of these devices,
the collimator has become the device of choice in most
imaging systems.

■ Collimation is a term used to describe the technique of
shaping the size of the x-ray beam to the area of interest being imaged.

■ A collimator consists of a series of adjustable metal
leaves and a light source to define the x-ray beam size
and shape used for the examination.

■ Collimation can be manual or automatic.

■ Radiation protection standards require that collimation
be used to ensure that the x-ray beam is the size of the
image receptor or smaller.

X-Ray Table

The x-ray table serves several functions, primarily to support
the weight of the patient. Several characteristic and significant
features of x-ray tables are listed.

■ Tabletops must be made of radiolucent materials so as not
to interfere with transmission of the beam onto the film. If
the tabletop absorbs too much of the beam, then the dose
to the patient would have to be increased to ensure that
the proper amount of radiation reaches the film.

■ Tabletops can be fixed, moving, and floating. A floating
tabletop implies that the top can be moved in any direction to facilitate patient positioning.

■ All tables should feature a Bucky assembly, which consists of a tray to hold the film cassette, a grid to prevent
scattered radiation from getting to the film, and a circuit
to move the grid so that grid lines will not be seen on the
film.

■ Accessories such as foot supports, hand grips, compression bands, head supports, and shoulder pads are useful devices to facilitate patient comfort and positioning.

Image Receptor

The image receptor for film-based radiography is a film-screen
cassette used to capture and record data from the patient. This
data is the x-ray beam transmitted through the patient. The

technologist must select the appropriate image receptor that meets the requirements of the examination. For example, if the detail of the bones of the extremities is of interest, then a "detail" cassette must be used.

Image receptors is described in greater detail later in this chapter.

Film Processing Equipment

When the transmitted beam of x-rays reaches the image receptor, a latent image is created on the film. To render this image visible, it must be processed by chemical means.

- The purpose of a film processing system (film processor) is to convert the latent image on the film to a visible image suitable for viewing by an observer.
- The image is rendered visible by subjecting the latent image on the film to a series of processing steps.
- These steps include wetting, developing, stop bath, fixing, washing, and drying.

Film processors can be manual or automatic. However, automatic processors have become state-of-the-art equipment in radiology departments since manual processors take too long to process film.

IMAGE RECEPTOR: FILM-BASED RADIOGRAPHY

The image receptor for film-based radiographic imaging systems includes the radiographic cassette, which holds the radiographic film.

The cassette consists of a pair of intensifying screens. When loading the cassette in the darkroom, the technologist places the film between the two screens. The purpose of the intensifying screens is to capture the radiation beam passing through the patient and convert the x-ray photons into light, a process referred to as luminescence. Intensifying screens in particular exhibit fluorescence (i.e., they emit light only when struck by x-rays). It is this light that forms the latent image on the film.

There are at least three elements of intensifying screens of practical importance to the technologist. These are the type of phosphor used, the characteristics of the phosphor, and the care and handling of the cassette.

Phosphor Materials

The phosphor is a significant component of the intensifying screen. The type of phosphor used determines how the cassette can meet the requirements of the various examinations.

- The phosphor converts the x-ray beam into light photons for creating the latent image. This is the conversion efficiency.
- The atomic number (number of protons in the nucleus) of the phosphor should be high to ensure greater absorption of the x-ray beam.
- Current phosphor materials are rare earth materials, including yttrium tantalate, lanthanum oxybromide, gadolinium oxysulfide, lanthanum oxysulfide, among others.
- Since different phosphors emit different colors of light (e.g., gadolinium oxysulfide emits green light, lanthanum oxybromide emits blue light), their spectral emission must match the film sensitivity (spectral matching).
- The thickness of the phosphor layer can range from 50 μm to 250 μm, and the size of the phosphor crystals can vary from 5 μm to 15 μm.

Characteristics of Intensifying Screens

When selecting an image receptor for a particular examination, the technologist must pay careful attention to several characteristics of the intensifying screen. These characteristics play an important role in establishing a trade-off between the amount of radiation used and the image quality desired. They include:

- *Screen sensitivity.* Screen sensitivity, or screen speed, is the amount of radiation required to produce an image.
  - ❏ Manufacturers use numbers to denote the speed (or relative exposure requirements), such as 100, 200, 400, 800, and 1000, and establish the screen speed. The reference speed is 100 and it is referred to as a par-speed system.
  - ❏ "Whereas sensitivity is a precise receptor characteristic that expresses the amount of exposure the receptor requires, speed is a less precise value used to compare film-screen combinations" (Sprawls, 1995).

❑ Sensitivity is inversely proportional to speed, which means that as the speed value is increased, the dose needed for the examination is decreased. For example, a 100-speed value has a sensitivity of 1.28 mR compared with 0.64 and 0.32 for 200- and 400-speed systems, respectively.

❑ The higher speed reduces radiation exposure, increasing the degradation in image quality (detail).

❑ Screen speed also depends on the absorption efficiency and the conversion efficiency of the screen.

■ *Absorption efficiency.* Absorption efficiency refers to the percentage of x-ray photons absorbed by the screen.

❑ As noted by Sprawls, "Absorption efficiency and screen sensitivity are highest when the x-ray photon energy is slightly above the K-edge of the absorbing material. Each intensifying screen material generally has a different sensitivity-photon energy relationship because its K-edge is at a different energy from the other materials" (1995).

❑ Screen sensitivity (speed) changes with kVp (photon energy), thus exposure factors (kVp and mAs) must be carefully adjusted depending on the sensitivity of the screen system in use.

■ *Conversion efficiency.* Conversion efficiency refers to the ability of the screens to convert the absorbed x-ray photons into light photons for image formation on the film. "With fixed absorption efficiency, changes in conversion efficiency are the greatest contributor to the change in image receptor speed" (Bushong, 2001).

■ *Image definition or detail.* The detail that an intensifying screen can generate depends on the phosphor size, thickness of the phosphor layer, and film-screen contact. Although smaller crystals and thinner phosphor layers will produce better resolution (detail), poor film-screen contact will result in poor resolution (image is blurred in the areas of poor contact).

■ *Noise.* A noisy image is formed by a limited amount of x-ray photons. Image noise appears as graininess or is mottled in appearance (quantum mottle of the image).

Increasing the number of photons reaching the film demands an increase in the mAs. Increasing the mAs, however, increases the dose. An increase in kVp with an appropriate adjustment of the mAs can produce sufficient photons to reduce image noise and dose to the patient.

Film Structure and Characteristics

The x-ray film is an integral component of the image receptor. The film can have either a single- or double-emulsion coating on a polyester base.

- The emulsion contains grains of silver bromide mixed with silver nitrate and potassium bromide. Latent image formation is as a result of the interaction of light from the intensifying screens with the crystal grains.
- Until recently, emulsion grains were three-dimensional in shape. However, modern x-ray films now feature grains that are tabular and cubic in shape.
  - ❏ Although tabular grains improve image sharpness, they produce a lower overall contrast, since grains deeper in the emulsion receive less exposure.
  - ❏ Cubic grains, conversely, produce higher contrast and are commonly used in laser imaging films and mammography films.

X-ray film, as in intensifying screens, has a number of characteristics of relevance to the technologist. These include:

- *Speed.* The speed of a film is its sensitivity, which relates to the amount of radiation exposure required to produce an image. Films can have a high sensitivity, in which case they require less exposure compared with films that have a low sensitivity. The choice of film speed depends on the nature of the examination. Although high-speed films reduce patient dose and the heat loading of the x-ray tube, low-speed films reduce image noise.
- *Spectral sensitivity.* This characteristic is important and must be considered when using intensifying screens and imaging cameras. Knowing the color of light emitted by the different types of intensifying screens is vital. The film response must match the color of light given off by the screen. This is referred to as spectral imaging. If, for example, a screen emits blue-green light, then the film

must be sensitive to this light for optimal image quality. Additionally, if a laser is used to write the image onto the film, then that film must be sensitive to the color of the laser beam.

■ *Contrast.* Film contrast refers to differences in density values on the film. The film converts the information contained in the radiation beam after it passes through the patient (subject contrast) into film contrast.

❑ Film contrast is determined by the slope of the characteristic curve, also referred to as the Hurter and Driffield (H and D) curve. The purpose of the characteristic curve is to demonstrate how much contrast a film will produce for a wide exposure range.

❑ The characteristic curve has three regions: the toe, shoulder, and a region in between the toe and shoulder, the region of maximum contrast or slope. While the toe region indicates low or light density (i.e., little or no contrast), the shoulder region indicates dark areas with reduced contrast. The slope (average gradient) of the curve provides optimal contrast.

■ *Latitude.* Latitude refers to the exposure range that results in optimal contrast. A wide exposure latitude film can tolerate an exposure error of approximately 15%. This characteristic decreases repeat films, thus the dose to the patient.

■ *Reciprocity law.* For nonscreen films, the exposure is directly proportional to the intensity of the beam and time of the exposure. This is the reciprocity law and it does not hold true for films that are used with intensifying screens. Reciprocity law failure occurs with extremely short or extremely long exposure times.

Film Processing

The latent image is created when x-rays fall on the silver-halide grains of the film. These grains exposed to x-rays are developed using a special chemical solution containing a variety of chemicals. The unexposed grains are removed from the emulsion through a chemical process called fixing. The latent image is now rendered visible and is permanently recorded on the film.

TABLE 2-1	Chemicals Found in the Developer of an X-Ray Film Processor	
COMPONENT	CHEMICAL	FUNCTION
Developing agent	Phenidone	Reducing agent; produces shades of gray rapidly
Developing agent	Hydroquinone	Reducing agent; produces black tones slowly
Buffering agent	Sodium carbonate	Helps swell gelatin; produces alkalinity; controls pH
Restrainer	Potassium bromide	Antifog agent; keeps unexposed crystals from being chemically attacked
Preservative	Sodium sulfite	Controls oxidation; maintains balance among developer components
Hardener	Glutaraldehyde	Controls emulsion swelling; aids archival quality
Sequestering agent	Chelates	Removes metallic impurities; stabilizes developing agent
Solvent	Water	Dissolves chemicals for use

From Bushong S. Radiologic Science for Technologists. 6th ed. St. Louis: Mosby, 2001. Reproduced with permission.

Main Stages of Film Processing

Film processing in radiology, whether automatic or manual, consists of the following stages:

- **Development.** The first stage in film processing is development. This stage takes place in the developer, which contains a variety of components and chemicals intended to develop density on the film (Table 2-1).
  - Optimal development results in a film with proper contrast.
  - Under development results in a film with reduced contrast.
  - Over development results in a darker film having the same appearance as an over-exposed film.
- **Fixing.** The next stage in film processing is fixing. The fixer tank contains several chemicals that ensure that the image (from the development process) will be per-

TABLE 2-2	Chemicals Found in the Fixer of an X-Ray Film Processor	
COMPONENT	CHEMICAL	FUNCTION
Activator	Acetic acid	Neutralizes the developer and stops its action
Fixing agent	Ammonium thiosulfate	Removes undeveloped silver bromide from emulsion
Hardener	Potassium alum	Stiffens and shrinks emulsion
Preservative	Sodium sulfite	Maintains chemical balance
Buffer	Acetate	Maintains proper pH
Sequestering agent	Boric acid and salts	Removes aluminum ions
Solvent	Water	Dissolves other components

From Bushong S. Radiologic Science for Technologists. 6th ed. St. Louis: Mosby, 2001. Reproduced with permission.

manent on the film. These chemicals and their associated functions are listed in Table 2-2.

- *Washing.* The film then travels from the fixer tank to the wash tank that contains water to remove any fixer solution that may remain on the emulsion. If the hypo (thiosulfate) is not removed, it will react with the silver nitrate to produce yellowish-brown color on the film, thus degrading image quality.
- *Drying.* This is the final stage for the film as it is removed from the fixer tank. During this stage, hot air is blown over the film to remove any moisture.

RADIOGRAPHIC IMAGE QUALITY

One of the goals of a technologist when conducting an examination is to produce a film with optimal image quality. The characteristics of a film that determine its quality are resolution, contrast, noise, distortion, and artifacts (Sprawls, 1995).

Resolution

Resolution refers to a characteristic that allows an observer to view separate objects on a film. There are two types of resolution: spatial resolution and contrast resolution. The former refers to detail (or visibility of detail) and the latter refers to the differences in tissue contrast that can be viewed on the film.

■ *Spatial resolution* refers to detail and is measured in line pairs per millimeter (lp/mm). The greater number of lp/mm that a film can demonstrate provides increased detail.

■ *Detail* is affected by several factors, such as the size of the focal spot, the motion of the patient, and the characteristics of the image receptor. Detail is at its optimum when small focal spots are used, when the patient does not move during the exposure, and when detail cassettes are used.

Contrast

As mentioned earlier, contrast is a significant image quality characteristic and is the density differences on a radiograph. A high-contrast image is characterized by regions of higher density (dark) and lower density (light).

Several factors affect the contrast of a radiograph, including the object, energy of the beam, scattered radiation, grids, and the film.

■ The main controlling factor for contrast, however, is kVp. Optimal contrast is produced when low-kVp techniques are used, since the photoelectric effect predominates.

■ A grid improves radiographic contrast by absorbing scattered radiation before reaching the film.

Noise

When insufficient photons are used to create an image on x-ray film, the image will be noisy and have a grainy appearance (quantum mottle). Because the main controlling factor for the number of photons is mAs, lower mAs will result in more noise compared with high-mAs techniques. Additional factors affecting noise are high kVp and high-speed image receptors. High-kVp techniques will reduce noise (since more photons are produced and strike the film) and high-speed image receptors will increase noise (since they require few photons for the production of the image when compared with slower image receptors).

The technologist must therefore select the best possible factors to produce optimal image quality.

Distortion

Distortion of the image can result when certain relationships between the object and the imaging system (x-ray tube and image receptor) are not observed. For example, objects must be as close as possible to the image receptor to reduce the size distortion resulting from magnification. Additionally, examinations that require tube angulations always result in image distortion.

Artifacts

An artifact is something that appears on the image that is not present in the patient. Artifacts may arise from the patient (patient motion), from equipment (processor, patient table, grids), and from storage and handling of x-ray films. To produce films with optimal image quality, the technologist must be fully aware of the wide range of factors affecting image quality and the components of the equipment directly responsible for the production of the radiograph. Additionally, the technologist must realize that there is a trade-off between image quality and dose to the patient. Every effort should be made to optimize the examination techniques to ensure the best possible image.

X-Ray Generators

Chapter at a glance

The x-ray generator is described briefly in terms of a few basic components, such as transformers and rectifiers, in Chapter 2. The purpose of the x-ray generator is to provide electrical energy, not only to the x-ray tube, but also other parts of the machine; thus the operator has full control of x-ray production.

In this chapter, the generator is described in detail. First, the functional characteristics of the generator are outlined, after which a description of three types of generators and their associated voltage waveforms are presented. The third major topic addresses the major components of the generator. The chapter concludes with a discussion of high-frequency generators and the power rating of a generator.

A firm understanding of the x-ray generator will provide the technologist with the tools to select and control the x-ray beam energy (quality), quantity, and the exposure time appropriate to the examination. Additionally, the technologist will be able to protect the patient from unnecessary radiation and the x-ray tube from possible electrical overload.

PURPOSE OF THE X-RAY GENERATOR

The basic generator circuit is made up of several subsystems that are interconnected to provide selection and control of various parameters for both radiographic and fluoroscopic examinations (Figure 3-1). The components include the high-voltage circuit, stator circuit, filament circuit, automatic exposure and brightness control circuits, focal spot selector, and density control.

The functions of an x-ray generator are to:

- Allow the operator to select and control the kilovolts peak (kVp) and milliamperage (mA) and time in seconds (mAs) necessary for the examination.
- Allow the operator to select the focal spot size appropriate to the requirements of the examination.
- Allow the operator a choice of manual or automatic exposure timing.

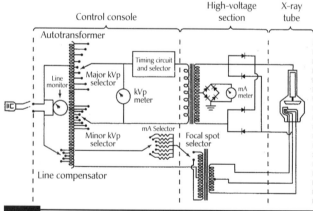

Figure 3-1 Electrical circuit diagram of an x-ray generator in its most basic form. The circuit can be divided into three parts for simplicity: the operating console or primary side, the high voltage section, and the x-ray tube. (*From Bushong S. Radiologic science for technologists. St. Louis: Mosby, 2001. Reproduced with permission.*)

- Increase the low voltage from the utility company to high voltage (kilovolts [kVs]) necessary for x-ray production.
- Decrease the high current from the utility company to milliamperage (mA) that determines the quantity of x-rays from the x-ray tube.
- Convert the alternating current (AC) from the utility company to direct current (DC) required by the x-ray tube to allow electrons to flow from the cathode to the anode.
- Protect the x-ray tube from any combination of kVp and mAs applied to the focal spot that may result in an electrical overload situation.
- Protect the operator and patient from electrical shock from the high voltage involved when using the x-ray machine.
- Prevent the x-ray tube from reaching its heat loading capacity, especially in examinations requiring a series of exposures, such as interventional angiography procedures.
- Protect the patient from unnecessary radiation through fail-safe mechanisms incorporated into the circuitry to prevent exposure resulting from faulty automatic timers. For example, the back-up time per mAs is intended to serve this function.
- Protect the patient by allowing the operator to have full control of the parameters affecting both the quality and the quantity of the x-ray beam.
- Enable identification and speedy resolution of a generator problem through the use of a service module that is a part of the system.

X-Ray Generator Circuit

The electrical circuit diagram for an x-ray generator in its most basic form (see Figure 3-1) can be divided into three sections:

- The *primary side of the circuit* (also referred to as the operating console) is the low-voltage side that allows the technologist to turn the machine on and off. This circuit also enables the operator to have full control of the parameters that affect the production of x-rays, image quality, and radiation dose to the patient.

■ The *secondary side of the circuit* (the high-voltage side),
which contains a number of components and the circuitry to provide the electrical power to the x-ray tube
that is required for x-ray production.

■ The characteristic features of the *x-ray tube* itself are
described in Chapter 4.

Power Supply to the Generator

The power supply to the x-ray generator from the electrical
utility company is alternating current (AC) with a frequency of
60 cycles per second or 60 Hertz (Hz).

■ 1 Hz = 1 cycle per second
■ 60 Hz = 60 cycles per second (low frequency)
■ 1 cycle per second = 2 impulses per second
■ 60 cycles per second = 120 (60 × 2) impulses per second

Two types of alternating current (AC) power supplies are
available:

■ *Single-phase AC power.* This power supply is produced by
a single-phase AC generator from the utility company
and has a single circuit. The circuit produces an AC
waveform that starts at 0 degrees (origin) in the positive
half cycle and reaches a maximum peak at 90 degrees,
then passes through 0 volts at 180 degrees, after which
it reverses polarity (negative half cycle) and reaches a
negative peak at 270 degrees and subsequently returns to
the origin (0 degrees) at 360 degrees. This cycle repeats
itself. The x-rays produced by a single-phase x-ray generator are low-energy and do not meet the requirements
of more sophisticated x-ray examinations requiring more
penetrating x-rays and shorter exposure times.

■ *Three-phase AC power.* A three-phase power supply
from the utility company has three separate AC input
lines producing three separate waveforms that have the
same frequency and voltage amplitude. Rather than
being in-phase with each other, however, they are out
of phase by one-third of a cycle or by 120 degrees. X-
ray production using a three-phase generator is substantially more efficient compared with a single-phase
generator. Greater tube output and shorter exposure
times are possible.

Primary Side of the Generator Circuit

The following basic components are found on the primary or low-voltage circuit of generator circuit:

- *On-off switch.* This switch allows the operator to turn the machine on before imaging the patient and off after use.
- *Line voltage compensator.* Automatic voltage compensation ensures that the correct input voltage is available to the entire circuit in the event of power variations in the hospital. The incorrect line or supply voltage can affect the output beam from the x-ray tube and, consequently, can have an effect on image quality. The line voltage compensator ensures that the machine receives precisely 220 volts (see Figure 3-1).
- *Autotransformer.* The input line voltage is delivered to an autotransformer that consists of a single electrical winding to provide the appropriate voltage to the high-voltage circuit, including the filament transformer. The autotransformer:
  - ❏ Has primary connections to accommodate the input power (shown on the left side of Figure 3-1).
  - ❏ Has secondary connections (on the right side of Figure 3-1) to provide the required voltage to other parts of the circuit.
  - ❏ Increases the input voltage by a factor of 2. The autotransformer can also decrease the voltage as well.
  - ❏ Works on the principle of electromagnetic induction and is based on the following law referred to as the autotransformer law:

  $$\frac{\text{Secondary voltage, V}_s}{\text{Primary voltage, V}_p} = \frac{\text{Number of secondary windings, N}_s}{\text{Number of primary windings, N}_p}$$

- *kVp selector and meter.* The kVp is an exposure factor that affects the penetrating power of the beam and can be selected in large (major) or small (minor) increments. The selector is connected to the autotransformer (see Figure 3-1). The voltage selected at this point by the technologist is the input voltage to the high-voltage transformer. The kVp meter, conversely, is a prereading voltmeter, and because it is positioned across the autotransformer lines (see Figure 3-1), it measures the voltage and not the kVp to the x-ray tube. On the control console, however, the kVp meter shows the kV that will be applied to the x-ray tube.

- **Filament circuit.** This circuit consists of the filament transformer, mA selector, and the focal spot selector. The circuit determines the filament current (approximately 3 to 6 amperes), which affects the tube mA. The mA is the main controlling factor for the quantity of photons from the x-ray tube and is controlled by the filament circuit. The autotransformer provides the voltage to the filament circuit through precision resistors (mA selector). "The filament transformer is a step-down transformer; therefore the voltage supplied to the filaments is lower, by a factor equal to the turns ratio, than the voltage supplied to the filament transformer. Similarly, the current is increased across the filament transformer in proportion to the turns ratio" (Bushong, 2001). The focal spot selector allows the technologist to select either a large or small focal spot size appropriate to the requirements of the examination.

- **Exposure timer.** Exposure timer is a manual or automatic electronic timer that determines the length of the exposure (beam-on time) in seconds (s). The product of mA and (s) is the mAs, which is also a controlling factor for the quantity of photons from the x-ray tube. Because the exposure timer is an important tool for the technologist, it is described in detail in Chapter 6.

Secondary Side of the Generator Circuit

The secondary side of the generator circuit is also called the high-voltage side of the generator. As noted in Figure 3-1, the high-voltage side consists of the high-voltage transformer, rectifiers, the filament transformer, and the mA meter. The high-voltage generator (tank) contains the high-voltage transformer, rectifiers, and the filament transformer, all immersed in oil, which provides electrical insulation.

- **High-voltage transformer.** Because of the turns ratio (ratio of the number of secondary windings to primary windings), this step-up transformer increases the low-voltage (volts) input from the autotransformer to high voltage (kVs) required for x-ray production. The turns ratio is about 500:1 to 1000:1, thus the input voltage can be increased by approximately 500 to 1000 times.

❏ The input (low voltage) to the high-voltage transformer is AC because transformers operate with AC. The output voltage waveform (high voltage) is also AC, but with greater amplitude than the input waveform.

❏ As noted by Seibert, "The output of the high-voltage transformer is 'center-tapped' to ground. Consequently, the maximum potential difference created by the high-voltage transformer is divided evenly with respect to ground, where one half of the secondary potential difference is positive and the other half is negative at any point in time. Thus for 100,000 V, +50 kV exists on one pole of the transformer and −50 kV exists on the other pole. The overall potential difference between the poles is +50−(−50 kV)=100 kV. Relative to ground, however, the peak voltage is only one-half of the peak potential difference, which minimizes the electrical insulation safety requirements for high-voltage cables" (1997).

■ *Rectifiers.* Arranged systematically in a circuit called the rectifier circuit, rectifiers convert the AC from the high-voltage transformer into direct current (DC) because the x-ray tube requires DC for x-ray production. Voltage rectification is described further in the next section.

■ *Filament transformer.* This step-down transformer works with relatively low voltage and high current, or 10V and 5A respectively. The transformer allows the technologist to provide the appropriate power to the x-ray tube filament for electron emission. The filament current (A) determines the temperature of the filament, thus the number of electrons that will be available for bombarding the target of the x-ray tube. When the filament temperature is higher, the amount of electrons available and the quantity of x-rays emitted from the tube are greater.

■ The *mA meter,* which is located in the secondary circuit and is connected near the electrical ground (center) of the secondary winding of the high-voltage transformer, measures the tube current (mA), which is the flow of electrons across the x-ray tube during the exposure. This ensures electrical safety, and for this reason, the mA/mAs meter can be placed on the control console.

RECTIFIERS AND RECTIFICATION

Modern rectifiers are solid-state, semi-conducting materials, such as pure silicon, designed to allow electrons to flow only in one direction. In the x-ray tube, electrons must flow from cathode to anode.

- Rectification changes the AC high-voltage output from the step-up transformer into direct voltage and current to allow electrons to flow only from cathode to anode in the x-ray tube.
- A rectification circuit is a component of the high-voltage side of the generator and consists of a series of rectifiers arranged systematically (see Figure 3-1) to change AC to DC.
- Rectifiers can be valve or solid-state diodes. The x-ray tube itself can be considered a valve diode (because it contains two electrodes: an anode and a cathode). Electron flow in these diodes is always from the electron source (cathode) to the electron target (anode). A solid-state rectifier has a p–n junction to allow electrons to flow only in one direction (Figure 3-2).
- Rectification can be either half wave or full wave (Figure 3-3). This circuit is a bridge rectifier circuit that illustrates how the rectifiers are arranged to ensure that electron flow is always from cathode to anode of the x-ray tube, independent of the high-voltage transformer polarity.

Half-Wave Rectification

Half-wave rectification is no longer used in modern radiology departments because this type of circuit uses only the positive half of the AC waveform for x-ray production. The negative half of the AC waveform is not used and is therefore wasted. X-rays are produced in pulses for a total of 60 pulses per second. Therefore x-ray output is limited with half-wave rectifier circuitry.

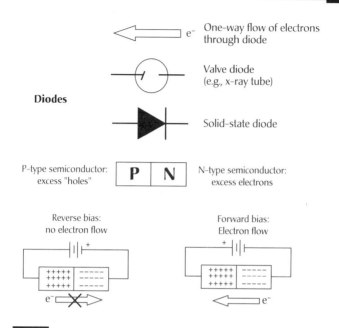

One-way flow of electrons through diode

Valve diode (e.g., x-ray tube)

Solid-state diode

Diodes

P-type semiconductor: excess "holes"

| P | N |

N-type semiconductor: excess electrons

Reverse bias: no electron flow

Forward bias: Electron flow

Figure 3-2 Circuit diagram symbols for valve and solid-state diodes. Electron flow is from the source of electrons to the electron target. In the bottom diagram, electrons flow only when a forward bias is applied and travel from negative to positive through the P-N junction. *(From Seibert A: X-ray generators.* Radiographics *17:1533, 1997. Reproduced with permission.)*

Full-Wave Rectification

Full-wave rectification overcomes this limitation by using the negative half of the AC waveform for x-ray production (see Figure 3-3). Four rectifiers are now used in this circuit to ensure that electron flow through the x-ray tube (for both the positive and negative portions of the AC waveform) is always from cathode to anode. X-rays now produce 120 pulses per second rather than at 60 pulses per second (for half-wave rectification). Full-wave rectified units produce x-rays more efficiently with shorter exposure times.

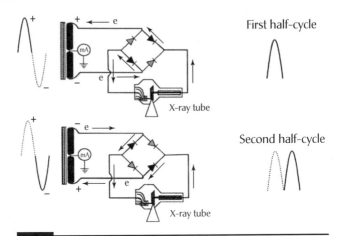

First half-cycle

Second half-cycle

Figure 3-3 Diagram illustrates the flow of electrons through a bridge rectifier circuit during each half-cycle of the applied voltage. The group of diodes is arranged so that the electron flow is always diverted through the cathode to the anode of the x-ray tube, independent of the change in polarity of the high-voltage transformer. For each half-cycle, two of the four diodes conduct (black diodes symbols). *(From Seibert A: X-ray generators,* Radiographics *17:1533, 1997. Reproduced with permission.)*

TYPES OF X-RAY GENERATORS

There are several types of x-ray generators based on their design complexity and cost. These generators include the single-phase generator (see Figure 3-1), the three-phase generator, the constant potential generator, and the high-frequency generator. Each of these generator types consists of the basic components previously described (see Figure 3-1). However, they differ in the efficiency with which they produce x-rays. Each generator type produces a characteristic voltage waveform or ripple (to be described subsequently) and x-ray beam spectra (quality and quantity of photons).

In this section, only the essential characteristics of three-phase and high-frequency generators are highlighted, because they are the most common in radiology departments.

Voltage Ripple

The voltage ripple is the voltage variation per cycle, and it "describes the percentage difference between the minimum and maximum voltages divided by the maximum voltage in the circuit" (Seibert, 1997).

$$\% \text{ voltage ripple} = \frac{V_{max} - V_{min}}{V_{max}} \times 100$$

where V_{max} = maximum voltage
V_{min} = minimum voltage

- A single-phase generator has the highest ripple or 100%, which explains why it is limited in its radiation output (beam quantity and quality) and produces higher radiation dose to patients with poorer image quality compared with other generators.
- A voltage ripple of 100% means that the voltage going to the x-ray tube varies from zero to some maximum value, the peak of the waveform. As a result, x-rays are produced using a wide range of voltages, that is, low to high (peak). Therefore the x-ray intensity varies from low-intensity (for low voltages) to high-intensity (as the peak voltage is reached). This factor means that the patient absorbs low energy x-rays because they have insufficient energy to reach the film. It is logical then to produce x-rays at peak voltages, thus the "p" (peak) in kVp.
- A ripple of 13% means that the voltage to the x-ray tube begins at 87% of the maximum value and never falls below 87% of the maximum value.
- A ripple of 3% means that the voltage to the x-ray tube never falls below 97% of the maximum value. This value results in higher radiation output (beam quality and quantity), less radiation dose to the patient, and the use of shorter exposure times.

Three-Phase Generators

The goal of designing and building better generators is to reduce the voltage ripple. A generator with the lowest voltage ripple implies that it provides the most efficient way to produce x-rays.

Three-phase generators overcome the limitations of single-phase generators by producing voltage waveforms with low ripple. This characteristic has implications for exposure technique factors. Bushong, for example, points out, "Three-phase operation may require as much as a 10 kVp reduction to produce the same radiographic optical density when operated at the same mAs as single-phase. A 12 kVp reduction may be necessary when using a high-frequency generator. Three-phase radiographic equipment is manufactured with tube currents as high as 1200 mA; therefore exceedingly short, high-intensity exposures are possible" (2001).

Two types of three-phase generators are available:

- *Three-phase, six-pulse generator*, which has six rectifiers to produce a voltage waveform with about 13% ripple. This generator produces six pulses per $\frac{1}{60}$ of a second compared with two pulses for a single-phase generator.
- *Three-phase twelve-pulse generator*, which has 12 rectifiers to produce an output waveform with approximately 4% ripple.
- *Three-phase generators* produce about a 12% increase in kVp or twice the mAs compared with single-phase generators.

High-Frequency Generators

The high-frequency generator is a state-of-the-art generator for use in radiology. The characteristic features of the essential components of a high-frequency generator (Figure 3-4) are:

- Low-frequency (60 Hz), low-voltage from the utility company is converted into a high-frequency (500 Hz to 25,000 Hz), low-voltage waveform and subsequently to a high-frequency, high-voltage output waveform that travels to the x-ray tube. The waveform to the x-ray tube is almost constant, with a ripple of less than 3%, resulting in a more efficient method of x-ray production with an increase in both x-ray intensity and beam energy (Figure 3-5).
- The high-frequency generator can use either a single-phase or a three-phase power supply. However, the three-phase input lines produce increased power.

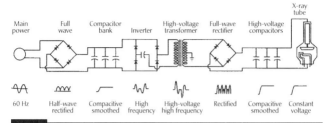

Figure 3-4 The essential circuit elements of a high-frequency generator showing the transformation of the voltage waveform on its way to the x-ray tube. *(From Bushong S. Radiologic science for technologists. 7th ed. St. Louis: Mosby, 2001. Reproduced with permission.)*

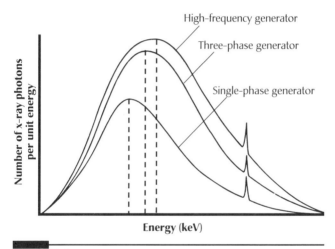

Figure 3-5 The intensity and effective beam energy produced by three types of generators. See text for further explanation. *(From Seeram E: Radiation protection, Philadelphia, 1997, Lippincott. Reproduced with permission.)*

- The high-frequency, high-voltage output from the high-voltage transformer is first rectified and subsequently smoothed by high-voltage capacitors to produce nearly constant voltage to the x-ray tube (see Figure 3-4).
- Autotransformers and space charge compensation circuits are not used because of closed-loop regulation cir-

cuits. These circuits ensure accurate kVp and mA linearity, as well as technique reproducibility and accurate exposure timing.

■ High-frequency generators are compact and can also be used in portable x-ray units and in modern CT scanners. These generators are inexpensive and can be easily serviced because of their use of microprocessor technology to facilitate maintenance.

■ Because of its high x-ray output (beam quality and quantity), a high-frequency generator delivers less radiation dose to the patient for a particular examination, compared with single- and three-phase generators (see Figure 3-5).

■ High-voltage capacitors are located in between the rectifiers and the x-ray tube to help provide a constant voltage to the tube. "As the voltage rises towards its peak, electrons from the rectifier circuit flow to both the x-ray tube and into the capacitor. When the voltage from the rectifier circuit begins to fall, electrons flow out of the capacitor and into the x-ray tube" (Sprawls, 1995).

POWER RATING OF AN X-RAY GENERATOR

The power rating of an x-ray generator takes into consideration the input voltage, the high voltage, and the filament transformer.

■ Power = amperes × volts (for constant current and voltage).

■ The unit of power is the watt (W).

■ The power rating of an x-ray generator is given in kilowatts (kW).

■ The power rating of a single-phase generator is:

$$\text{Power rating (kW)} = \frac{\text{mA} \times \text{kVp}}{1000} \times 0.7$$

Because of the high voltage ripple, the rating is reduced by approximately 30%.

■ The power rating of a three-phase generator is:

$$\text{Power rating} = \frac{\text{mA} \times \text{kVp}}{1000}$$

The power requirements for an x-ray generator should be based on the requirements of the particular clinical applications. Additionally, the power rating should be in terms of the focal spot size required for the application. A larger focal spot will have a higher power rating compared with a small focal spot size.

■ General radiographic imaging generators commonly have power ratings ranging from 30 kW to 50 kW.

■ Angiography and interventional imaging applications generally require generator power ratings equal to or less than 150 kW.

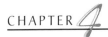
X-Ray Tubes for Diagnostic Radiology

Chapter at a glance

The x-ray tube produces a radiation beam best suited to the requirements of the examination and the desired quality of the image. The characteristics of the x-ray beam, such as the energy spectrum and the effective focal spot size, are influenced by the design of the x-ray tube and therefore by its major components.

The purpose of this chapter is to outline and review the major components of the x-ray tube, including variations in x-ray tube design and the heat capacity of x-ray tubes.

These topics are important to the technologist for several reasons:

- The x-ray tube is a vital tool that is used in all examinations.
- The x-ray beam characteristics affect image quality, such as spatial resolution (detail) and contrast, as well as patient dose.
- Several factors determine the conditions under which the tube can be operated safely for all examinations.
- Consideration of these factors will help extend the life of the tube.

PRODUCTION OF X-RAYS

X-rays are produced when high-speed electrons from the filament of the cathode (negative electrode) strike the target region of the anode (positive electrode).

X-Ray Generator

The x-ray generator (see Chapter 3) provides electrical energy to the x-ray tube for the production of x-rays. The generator also allows the technologist to select and control the energy of the beam (kilovolts peak [kVp]), the quantity of x-rays in the beam (milliamperage [mA]), and the length of time x-rays are produced (exposure time in seconds).

- The generator ensures that high voltage, ranging from 20 to 150 kVp, is applied between the cathode and the anode of the x-ray tube. This high voltage is responsible for accelerating electrons from cathode to anode at high speeds.
- The generator also provides the appropriate voltage waveform to the x-ray tube. The type of waveform determines the quality and quantity of the radiation beam emanating from the x-ray tube.
- The generation and production of x-rays is an inefficient process, meaning that, of the energy supplied to the x-ray tube, only 1% is converted into x-rays and 99% is converted into heat.

- The radiation produced by the tube is bremsstrahlung (brems) radiation, as well as characteristic radiation. Brems radiation is produced when electrons decelerate because of the force field of the nucleus. Characteristic radiation, conversely, is produced when electrons from the filament of the cathode interact with electrons in the inner shell of the x-ray tube target atom.
- Diagnostic radiology uses more brems radiation compared with characteristic radiation in most imaging examinations.

X-Ray Tube Requirements

To produce x-rays efficiently and to meet the criteria for optimizing image quality with reduced dose to the patient, an x-ray tube must be designed to provide:

- Extremely sharp images (high spatial resolution).
- Short exposure times to image moving structures without blurring resulting from motion.
- Capability for withstanding large electrical loads (kVp, mA, and time).
- Proper energy spectrum that is appropriate to the requirements of the examination. For example, a low-kVp technique will produce soft x-rays (low energy and less penetrating) required to image soft tissues.
- Rapid heat dissipation.

The remainder of this chapter explores the design features and components of the x-ray tube that meet the previously described requirements.

COMPONENTS OF X-RAY TUBES

The essential components of an x-ray tube include the cathode assembly, anode assembly, rotor and stator, tube envelope, and x-ray tube housing (Figure 4-1).

Cathode Assembly

The major components of the cathode assembly are a filament positioned in a metal cup, called a focusing cup.

- The filament is the source of electrons. It is made of tungsten wire wound in a helical coil (10 to 20 mm long and

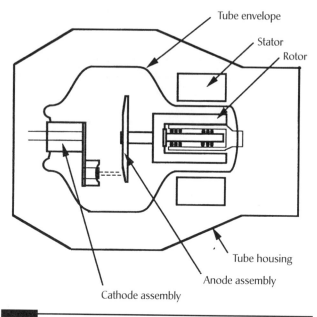

Figure 4-1 The essential components of an x-ray tube used in diagnostic radiology. *(From Zink FE. X-ray tubes. Radiographics 1997; 17:1259. Used with permission.)*

2 to 5 mm thick) to increase its surface area. Tungsten is used because of its high melting point (3410° C), and its high atomic number (Z = 74).

- The filament is heated via the filament circuit of the generator with approximately 3 to 6 amps to "boil-off" electrons by thermionic emission.

- With prolonged use, tungsten may vaporize and cause a build up in the inside of the envelope. This disturbs the electrical balance in the tube, the result of which may produce arcing. This tungsten vaporization is the most common cause of tube failure (Bushong, 2001).

- To prolong the life of the tube, tungsten filaments are coated with a layer of thorium (thoriated-tungsten filaments), thus the efficiency of thermionic emission is much greater compared with pure tungsten filaments.

- Most x-ray tubes are provided with two filaments positioned in the focusing cup: a large filament and a small filament. Although the large filament is used for examinations requiring a high-output intensity in a short time (e.g., abdomen, chest), the smaller filament is preferred when detail is important.
- The focusing cup has a negative charge and plays a role in focusing the electrons from the filament to strike the anode on a region called the target or focal spot.
- Power dissipation from the filament is approximately 40 watts (current [4 amp] × voltage [10 V]).
- The flow of electrons from cathode to anode is the tube current or mA. Electrons flow only when there is a potential difference (kV) between cathode and anode. The x-ray beam from the tube is directly proportional to the mA. Doubling the mA increases the quantity of photons by a factor of two. Doubling the mA also increases the patient dose by a factor of 2.
- Radiographic mA can range from 50 mA to 1000 mA, and the range for fluoroscopic mA is approximately 0.1 mA to 3.0 mA for modern units.

Anode Assembly

Anodes can be stationary or they can be rotating. There are several elements of the anode that play a role in the efficiency of x-ray production, image quality, heatloading, and heat dissipation (heat capacity).

- The stationary anode is made of a copper block in which a rectangular piece of tungsten is embedded. The tungsten is the target. The copper block conducts heat away from the tungsten target. Another characteristic of importance is that the face of the anode is inclined at an angle, called the target angle, to direct the radiation beam to the patient.
- Inclining the anode at specified angles leads to a design referred to as the line focus principle. This principle ensures a large area for heating and a small effective focal spot size. The effective focal spot is the focal spot projected onto the film. When the target angle is small, the effective focal spot size is also small, and the spatial

resolution (detail) of the image is better. X-ray tubes have target angles ranging from 5 to 15 degrees. As the target angle is increased, the field coverage at the image receptor is greater.

■ The line focus principle gives rise to the heel effect, during which the x-ray beam intensity along the anode-cathode axis varies. The relative intensity is 100% at the cathode side and decreases to approximately 50% at the anode side. This variation in intensity is a result of the fact that because x-rays are produced inside the target, the x-rays leaving the target at the anode side have to travel a longer distance through the target and are therefore absorbed, lowering the intensity at the anode side.

■ All x-ray tube anodes have a focal spot, a defined area on the target that electrons from the filament strike when they are accelerated from the cathode to the anode. This focal spot is called the actual focal spot. Tubes have both large and small focal spot sizes. When the focal spot size is smaller, the spatial resolution of the image is better. Larger focal spot sizes can withstand greater electrical loads (kVp, mA and time in seconds [mAs]) and have higher heat capacities compared with smaller focal spots. For example, higher mA and short exposure times can be safely used with large focal spots.

■ Stationary anode tubes are limited in their x-ray output (intensity) and heat loading. These tubes are suitable for applications that require only a low x-ray output, such as dental radiography and portable fluoroscopy.

These limitations are overcome by the rotating anode x-ray tubes.

The rotating anode is a disk supported by a molybdenum stem (see Figure 4-1). The fundamental features of the disk are as follows:

■ The diameter of the disk affects the maximum permissible load (kVp, mAs) that the tube can withstand. The diameter varies and can range from 50 to 200 mm. The larger diameter increases the exposure technique factors that the tube can withstand. Because the electron beam strikes a larger target area, the heat capacity of the tube increases.

- Earlier tubes used a pure tungsten disk. However, current state-of-the-art x-ray tubes use a compound anode disk.
- A compound anode disk is made of two or more metals and consists of a base body onto which a coating layer (layer bombarded by the electron beam) is deposited. These materials include rhenium (R), zirconium (Z), and titanium (T) used in conjunction with tungsten (T), molybdenum (M), and graphite. A typical compound anode is the Rhenium-Tungsten-Molybdenum (RTM) disk with molybdenum and/or graphite as the base, with 10% rhenium and 90% tungsten (coating layer).
- Compound anode disks have several advantages compared with pure tungsten disks.
  - ❏ Lesser rotational problems because of the lighter weight
  - ❏ Extreme resistance to the aging process
  - ❏ Greater heat storage capacity
  - ❏ Less roughening of the target track
  - ❏ A high and uniform dose over the entire life of the tube
  - ❏ Higher exposure technique factors (with shorter exposure times) can be used
- Target materials for x-ray tubes should have a high atomic number (Z), high thermal conductivity, and high melting point. The efficiency of x-ray production is directly proportional to Z. Higher Z materials produce x-rays more efficiently compared with lower Z materials.
- Rotating anode disks also feature two focal spot sizes (large and small) and have target angles that vary from 5 to 15 degrees. In addition, these anodes are also subject to the anode heel effect.

Rotation of the Anode Disk

An induction motor that consists of a stator and a rotor produces the rotation of the anode disk (see Figure 4-1).

- The purpose of rotating the disk is to increase the instantaneous heat load on the target (thereby increasing the x-ray output by increasing the effective surface area of the target).

- The induction motor produces the rotation speed of the disk and depends on the frequency of main supply to the stator. Typical speeds are approximately 3600 revolutions per minute (rpm). Increasing the rotation speed increases the heat capacity of the tube. Tubes with high-speed anode rotation rotate at 10,000 rpm.

- The induction motor consists of the stator that contains electrical windings to provide the force for anode rotation and the rotor, or "a shaft made of bars of copper and soft iron fabricated into one mass" (Bushong, 2001).

- Free and smooth rotation of the disk are made possible through the use of steel ball bearings lubricated with metallic barium, silver, or lead; ordinary lubricants reduce friction in the rotor assembly. Ball-bearing technology may result in mechanical problems from heating and cooling. To overcome this problem, a liquid-bearing method is now used in current state-of-the-art, high-capacity x-ray tubes, especially x-ray tubes used in computed tomography (CT).

- With liquid-bearing technology, the fixed shaft of the anode consists of grooves that contain gallium-based, liquid metal alloy. During anode rotation, the liquid is forced into the grooves, which causes a hydroplaning effect between the sleeve and the liquid. This technology conducts heat away from the disk more efficiently than ball-bearing technology. Additionally, the liquid bearing technology is free of noise and vibrations.

- As pointed out by the notable physicist Stewart Bushong, "When the operator pushes the exposure button of the radiographic unit, there is a one second wait before taking an exposure. This allows the rotor to accelerate to its designed revolutions per minute. During this time, filament current is increased to provide the correct x-ray tube current. When using a two-position exposure switch, it is important for the radiographer to push the switch to its final position in one motion. That minimizes the time that the filament is heated, which prevents excessive space charge and thus prolongs tube life" (2001).

X-Ray Tube Envelope

The envelope (also referred to as the tube insert) of an x-ray tube is an important component that serves several functions:

- Supports the internal components (anode and cathode structures) of the tube.
- Maintains a vacuum; any gas molecules in the tube will impede the flow of electrons from the cathode to anode. The gas may also cause oxidization of the filament and result in tube failure.
- All tube envelopes have an exit window or port (through which x-rays leave the tube) that is thinner than the envelope itself. This port filters the beam (inherent filtration) as it exits the tube.
- X-ray tube envelopes can be glass, glass and metal, or completely metal. High-capacity x-ray tubes have full metal envelopes. The problems with glass envelopes are limited heat storage capacity and less efficient heat dissipation, because metal deposits seriously affect the physical properties of glass. These problems are overcome with metal envelopes. Recent x-ray tubes have been designed with glass and metal envelopes and with full metal envelopes.
- The glass and metal envelope tube is a rotating anode x-ray tube having the same features described earlier, with a few notable differences.
  - ❏ The envelope consists of two glass end pieces with a central metal envelope.
  - ❏ The metal envelope encases the electric field between the cathode and anode and is not affected by tungsten deposits, compared with glass envelopes.
  - ❏ Higher tube currents and shorter exposure times can be used.
  - ❏ Two windows are provided: a beryllium window followed by an aluminum window.
  - ❏ A large volume anode disk is a characteristic feature of the glass and metal x-ray tube. The size of this disk allows the technologist to use higher exposure technique factors (with shorter exposure times), increases heat storage capacity, and allows for more efficient heat dissipation.

X-Ray Tube Housing

The envelope of the x-ray tube is encased in a protective housing called the tube housing or tube shield. The housing is cylindrical in shape and has two receptacles to accommodate the high-voltage cables from the generator.

- The purpose of the tube housing is to provide mechanical support for the insert, radiation shielding (ray-proofing), and electrical insulation.
- Oil is placed between the envelope and the inner walls of the housing to insulate and protect the housing from the high voltage applied to the tube and to facilitate heat dissipation.
- The housing is lined internally with thin sheets of lead to prevent radiation from "leaking" through the housing (ray-proofing). The protection guidelines for the housing requires that the housing must reduce the leakage radiation to less than 26 µC/kg − hour (100 mR/hr), 1 meter from the x-ray tube.

METAL-CERAMIC TUBE WITH DOUBLE BEARINGS

A recently introduced high-capacity rotating anode x-ray tube is the metal-ceramic tube with double bearings. The most important features in the design of this tube are the metal envelope, ceramic insulation, double-bearing axle, and the large anode disk.

Metal Envelope

The metal envelope ensures higher capacity, better mechanical stability, and better thermal and electrical properties than glass, making it suitable for use in angiography.

- The metal envelope is not susceptible to metal deposits from vaporization.
- The tube exit window features both beryllium and an interchangeable aluminum filter that can be changed to suit the requirements of the examination. Oil is also used to provide inherent filtration and electrical insulation.

Ceramic Insulation

Ceramic is bonded at both ends (cathode and anode) of the tube to ensure a tight vacuum seal.

- The purpose of using ceramic is to insulate the tube for voltages up to 150 kVp.
- Ceramic is also used at the rotor end of the anode and rotates with it and provides insulation of the disk and axle at high voltages.

Double-Bearing Axle

Conventional tubes have single-bearing axles to support the anode disk. The metal-ceramic tube, by virtue of its construction, can facilitate a larger disk than its counterparts. The disk is mounted onto a double-bearing axle. The purpose of this design is to ensure that the bearing load is more uniform (compared with conventional tubes). The benefit of this approach is to extend the life of the tube.

Disk

The disk for this type of tube is extremely large, approximately 200 mm in diameter. Larger disks provide improved cooling and the use of higher exposure technique factors (with shorter exposure times) compared with conventional tubes.

X-RAY TUBE HEAT CAPACITY

As stated earlier, when high-speed electrons strike the target, 1% of the energy supplied to the tube is converted into x-rays and 99% is converted into heat. The x-ray tube must be capable of handling this heat efficiently so that more exposures can be applied to the tube.

Understanding x-ray tube heat capacity warrants a brief description of heat loading, heat units, x-ray tube rating, and heat dissipation. These topics are important to the technologist since they play a vital role in preventing tube failure thus extending the life of the x-ray tube.

Heat Loading

The heat loading of an x-ray tube is defined as the amount of heat deposited during the application of one exposure.

Heat Unit

The heat unit (HU) is used to quantify the heat loading of an x-ray tube. A heat unit is the product of mA, kVp, exposure time, and a constant that depends on the type of generator (voltage waveform) used.

■ The HU for single-phase generators is given by:

$$HU_{single-phase} = kVp \times mA \times seconds$$

■ The HU for three-phase, 6-pulse generators is given by:

$$HU_{three-phase, 6 pulse} = kVp \times mA \times seconds \times 1.35$$

■ The HU for three-phase, 12-pulse generators is given by:

$$HU_{three-phase, 12-pulse} = kVp \times mA \times seconds \times 1.41$$

■ The heat capacity of a conventional anode is about 250,000 HU. The heat capacity is about 1,000,000 HU for larger state-of-the-art compound anodes.

X-Ray Tube Rating

Huda and Slone when discussing tube rating state, "The rating of an x-ray tube is based on maximum allowable kilowatts (kW) at an exposure time of 0.1 second. For example, a tube with a rating of 80 kW (80,000 W) tolerates a maximum exposure of 80 kVp, and 1000 mA at 0.1 second" (1995).

There are three tube rating charts that technologists need to understand: the radiographic rating chart, the anode cooling chart, and the x-ray tube housing cooling chart.

■ The *radiographic rating chart* provides data on the exposure technique factors (kVp, mA, time) that can be applied safely to the x-ray tube. If the factors are not safe, then the machine would automatically detect this and would prevent the technologist from taking the exposure.

❑ The chart is similar to a graph of kVp plotted as a function of time (in seconds) and a set of mA curves. A safe exposure would be read as a value below the appropriate mA curve for any combination of kVp and exposure time. Values above the curves are unsafe.

❑ When reading a chart, the technologist must pay attention to information on the chart such as the generator type, anode rotation speed, target angle, and focal spot size, to ensure that the correct chart is used.

- The *anode cooling chart* provides data on the heat capacity (HU) of the anode and the time required for a heated anode to cool (heat dissipation characteristics).
  - ❏ The chart provides data on the maximum anode heat-storage capacity, as well as the maximum anode cooling rate.
  - ❏ The cooling rate is the rate of heat dissipation of the anode when its temperature is at its maximum.
- The *x-ray tube housing cooling chart* provides data on the heat-storage capacity of the housing (because the heat from the anode is transferred to the housing via the oil in the housing), as well as the time required for the housing to cool. The chart is similar to the anode cooling chart and shows both the maximum heat-storage capacity (HU) and the total time required for the housing to cool completely.

Heat Dissipation

There are three processes by which heat is dissipated in the x-ray tube: conduction, convection, and radiation.

- Heat is transferred from the focal track to the anode body by conduction (energy transfer from one region to the next region of the object) and by radiation (emission of the infrared radiation) from the focal track to the tube housing.
- Heat is transferred from the anode body to the tube housing by radiation.
- Heat is transferred from the tube housing to the atmosphere in the room by convection. "The transfer of heat by movement of the heated object such as air, water, or oil from one place to another" (Bushong, 2001).

PREVENTING X-RAY TUBE FAILURE: PRACTICAL CONSIDERATIONS

There are several reasons why the x-ray tube may fail, but the more common ones under the direct control of the technologist are a single excessive exposure, the use of long exposure times, and high mA values.

To prevent x-ray tube failure, the technologist can do the following:

Single Excessive Exposure

Avoid using a single excessive exposure, which can cause the temperature of the anode to become excessively high and may result in melting and pitting the surface of the anode. Additionally, the tungsten may vaporize causing tungsten deposits in the glass envelope that can lead to electrical arcing. Excessively high anode temperatures may crack the anode, resulting in rotation problems.

A tube warm-up procedure can be used to prevent x-ray tube failure. This procedure can be accomplished when the tube has not been used for at least 45 minutes (Bushong, 2001) by making three exposures separated by 3 seconds each, using 200 mA, 80 kVp, and 1 second.

Long Exposure Times

Avoid using long exposure times (1 to 3 seconds) because the anode assembly heats excessively resulting in damage to the bearings, subsequently leading to rotational problems.

High mA Techniques

Avoid using high mA techniques. High mA use over extended periods tends to vaporize the filament, which leaves tungsten deposits on the glass envelope and may lead to electrical arcing. The filament becomes thinner and breaks (Bushong, 2001).

Radiographic Rating Charts

Always consult a radiographic rating chart for cases in which the safety of the exposure technique applied to the tube is in question. When exposing the patient using an exposure switch that has two positions (one for the rotor and one for the exposure), push the switch in one motion to reduce the filament heating time.

The x-ray tube is an important tool in imaging patients. This tool is used on a daily basis in radiography and fluoroscopy. Careful attention to the major components and principles of operation will ensure optimal image quality with reduced dose to patients and prolonged life of the x-ray tube.

Filtering the X-Ray Beam

Chapter at a glance

In radiography and fluoroscopy, the x-ray beam from the x-ray tube is a heterogeneous beam of radiation, as opposed to a homogeneous beam.

- In a homogeneous beam, all the photons have the same energy. That is, they all have the same wavelength.
- In a heterogeneous beam, the photons have different energies; that is, the beam is made up of long and short wavelength x-rays.

These long wavelength x-rays are low energy x-rays that have insufficient energy to penetrate the patient to reach the film and are therefore absorbed by the patient. This absorption results in an unnecessary increase in patient dose. It makes good sense then that if these low-energy x-rays can be removed from the beam, then the dose to the patient would be reduced. To accomplish this goal, a filter is used.

The purpose of this chapter is to review the various types of filters used in radiographic imaging systems and to highlight the effect of filtration on several imaging parameters such as patient dose and x-ray beam quantity and quality.

Knowledge of x-ray beam filtration is important to technologists because it provides them with an essential tool to minimize the radiation dose to the patient undergoing a radiologic examination.

What is a Filter?

A *filter* used in x-ray imaging systems is any material (usually a flat plate made of aluminum) to absorb, preferentially, low-energy rays from the x-ray beam.

- The process of absorbing low-energy photons, thus reducing the number of photons in the beam, is referred to as *filtration*.
- Filtration reduces patient dose and is always required in x-ray procedures.
- The filter is located near the x-ray tube and is always positioned between the tube and the patient.

Types of Filtration

As the beam leaves the target of the x-ray tube, it passes through several materials (including the patient) before it reaches the x-ray film. These materials include the envelope of the x-ray tube, the oil in the tube housing (outside the envelope), the exit window of the tube, and the added piece of metal outside the tube.

Two types of filtration are important to the technologist: inherent and added filtration.

Inherent Filtration

Inherent filtration is filtration from the glass envelope, oil, and the exit window of the x-ray tube.

- Inherent filtration is generally 0.5 mm aluminum equivalent.
- X-ray tubes designed for mammography occasionally have beryllium rather than glass as their exit window. Inherent filtration for these tubes is approximately 0.1 mm aluminum equivalent.

- Inherent filtration cannot be changed by the technologist.
- As the x-ray tube ages, tungsten may be deposited on the inside of the glass envelope resulting from vaporization of the tungsten filament. This build-up of tungsten deposit will increase the inherent filtration.

Added Filtration

An *added filter* is a sheet of aluminum close to the exit window of the x-ray tube. This point is also where the collimator is attached to the x-ray tube.

- The technologist has control of the amount of added filtration based on the kilovolts peak (kVp) used for the examination.
- The type and thickness of the added filter depends on the kVp being used. The higher the kVp, the thicker the filter.
- In most diagnostic radiography examinations, aluminum is the material of choice for added filtration.

During examinations that require high kVp techniques (above 100 kVp), a *compound filter* is often used. A compound filter is made of aluminum (at least 1 to 2 mm thick) and copper (at least 0.10 to 0.25 mm thick) with the copper positioned closer to the tube target. At high kilovoltages (kV), copper emits soft characteristic x-rays that are absorbed by the aluminum, which prevents these rays from reaching the patient. Aluminum also emits soft characteristic rays. However, these are absorbed by the air-gap between the x-ray tube and the patient. In some fluoroscopic equipment, the technologist can change the thickness of the filter, depending on the kVp requirements of the examination.

Total Filtration

The *total filtration* for radiographic imaging system is:

- Total filtration = inherent filtration + added filtration + filtration by the mirror of the collimator.
- Total permanent filtration must be as follows:
  - ❑ 0.5 mm aluminum equivalent below 50 kVp.
  - ❑ 1.5 mm aluminum equivalent for voltages between 50 kVp and 70 kVp.
  - ❑ 2.5 mm aluminum equivalent for voltages above 70 kVp.

EFFECTS OF FILTRATION ON X-RAY TUBE OUTPUT

The x-ray tube output can be described in terms of x-ray quantity and x-ray quality.

X-Ray Quantity

X-ray quantity is the number of x-ray photons in the beam of radiation emerging from the x-ray tube.

- Filtration reduces the beam quantity.
- Filtration reduces the optical density on the film.

X-ray quantity can also be referred to as radiation exposure. A filter reduces the dose to the patient by reducing the radiation exposure. To calculate the amount of reduction, the half-value layer (HVL) is used.

X-Ray Quality

The quality of an x-ray beam refers to the penetrating power or energy of the photons. As the energy increases, beam quality increases, as noted by Bushong:

- "The half-value layer of an x-ray beam refers to the thickness of absorbing material necessary to reduce the x-ray intensity to half its original value" (2001).
- The half-value layer characterizes the beam quality.
- Half-value layer for diagnostic x-rays is 3 to 5 mm of aluminum or 4 to 8 cm of soft tissue.
- Filtration increases beam quality because low-energy photons are selectively removed by the filter.
- As filtration increases, beam quantity decreases and beam quality (the mean energy of the photons) increases. This factor explains why filtration reduces patient dose and protects the patient from unnecessary radiation.
- The increase in the mean or effective energy of the beam is referred to as beam hardening.

HEAVY METAL FILTERS

Heavy elements such as gadolinium, iron, samarium, holmium, and tungsten have been used as filter materials in radiographic imaging, particularly in pediatric imaging.

- These filters play a significant role in skin dose reduction because they provide more attenuation compared with aluminum.
- A gadolinium filter (250 μm thick) provides better contrast than a 2 mm aluminum filter.

COMPENSATING FILTERS

A compensating filter is an accessory filter used in x-ray imaging systems to provide an even (uniform) distribution of film density when the object being imaged is of an uneven thickness, such as the foot or femur.

- A compensating filter works because "it compensates for differences in subject radiopacity" (Bushong, 2001).
- Compensating filters are manufactured in a wide variety of shapes and sizes to suit the requirements of a wide range of examinations.
- Compensating filters can be wedge-shaped, trough-shaped, bow-tie–shaped, conic-shaped, as well as the shape of a step-wedge. Examples of the use of these include the following:
  - ❏ Wedge filters are generally used when x-raying feet. The thick portion of the wedge is placed towards the patient's toes.
  - ❏ A bow-tie filter is used in computed tomography to make the beam more uniform at the detectors.

IMAGE DOSE DODGING

Image dose dodging or "dodging" is a technique developed in Sweden in the 1970s.

- The technique uses a series of compensating filters specially arranged not only to produce uniform film density, but also to enhance image quality and decrease the dose to the patient.
- One series of arrangements consists of a set of smoothly formed, adjustable aluminum wedges that can be adjusted to conform to the patient's anatomy under investigation.

- The entire dodging system can be attached to the collimator.
- The dodging system removes the "burnt-out" regions at the periphery of the radiograph thus improving the image allowing for better visualization of image details.
- Because the aluminum wedges absorbs the radiation falling on the periphery of the radiograph, unnecessary dose to the patient is eliminated.

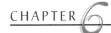

CHAPTER 6

Exposure Timers for Radiographic Systems

Chapter at a glance

One of the components of the x-ray generator is the exposure timing circuit. The exposure time is one of the main controlling factors affecting both radiographic density and radiation dose. In fact, the relationship between density and dose and exposure time is a direct proportionality. Doubling the exposure time will increase the density and dose by a factor of two.

All x-ray machines are equipped with exposure timers that allow the technologist to optimize the radiographic density while keeping the dose to the patient as low as reasonably achievable. The technologist can make a manual selection of the exposure time or an automatic exposure timer can be used.

This chapter outlines the principles of electronic exposure timers and automatic exposure control devices. These principles will provide the technologist with the skills needed to use the timer to its full potential while realizing its limitations.

LOCATION OF THE TIMER CIRCUITRY

As noted in Chapter 3 (see Figure 3-1), the exposure timing circuitry is located on the primary side of the generator circuit.

- Because the timer is positioned on the control console, it is maintained at low voltage to minimize the hazard of electrical shock.
- The circuit is positioned between the kilovolts peak (kVp) control and the primary side of the high-voltage transformer.

MAIN FUNCTION OF THE TIMER

The major purpose of the timer circuitry is:

- To determine the duration of the x-ray exposure or "beam-on" time by terminating the high-voltage between the anode and cathode. Only when this high-voltage is applied across the tube can electrons flow from cathode to anode to produce x-rays.
- The termination of the exposure is facilitated through the use of relays and mechanical contacts that act as switches in the circuitry.

TYPES OF EXPOSURE TIMERS

Several types of exposure timers have been developed for use in radiographic imaging systems. These include mechanical timers (now obsolete), synchronous timers (now obsolete), electronic timers (state-of-the-art technology) including the milliamperage/seconds (mAs) timer, and the automatic exposure timer. The electronic timer circuitry is a major component of automatic exposure timers. This chapter therefore focuses on the components and operation of the electronic timer.

Electronic Exposure Timer

As the notable radiological physicist Dr. Stewart Bushong points out, "Electronic timers are the most sophisticated, most complicated, and most accurate of the x-ray exposure timers" (2001).

The three major components of an electronic timer are a capacitor, a variable resistor, and a suitable switching device to "make" or "break" the high voltage applied between the cathode and anode of the x-ray tube. During operation of the timer, the capacitor must be charged to some critical value through the variable resistor. The time (t) for the capacitor to reach this critical value is directly proportional to (R) of the resistor times (C) of the capacitor, where

R = Resistance in ohms

C = Capacitance in farads

The product of R and C is known as the time constant of the circuit. As the R decreases, the exposure time for the examination shortens.

When the electronic timer is used in an examination, the technologist determines the exposure time best suited to the requirements of the examination. This may be a short exposure time (when patient motion is a problem) or a long exposure time (when a "breathing technique" is required). When an exposure is made, the following events occur:

- The capacitor begins to charge-up.
- The solid-state switching device (a silicon-controlled rectifier [SCR]) is activated ("on position") and the exposure begins.
- When the capacitor reaches its critical value, the SCR is turned off, and the exposure stops.
- The electronic timer can provide an exposure time as short as one millisecond (1 ms).

mAs Timer

The mAs timer may still be used in some x-ray machines. This timer is based fundamentally on the electronic timer. The technologist determines the mAs for the examination based on various imaging parameters. During the exposure:

- mA $\times$ time (mAs) are monitored by the timer.
- The exposure stops when the selected mAs is reached.
- "The mAs is usually designed to provide the highest safe tube current for the shortest time of exposure for any mAs selected. Since the mAs must monitor the actual

tube current, it is located on the secondary side of the high-voltage transformer" (Bushong, 2001).

Automatic Exposure Timers

Automatic exposure timing (phototiming) or automatic exposure control (AEC), to which it is often referred, is a system of exposure control or timing determined by the machine rather than the technologist. AEC was invented to overcome the problem of repeat exposures because of exposure timing errors imposed by manual selection of exposure times. The purpose of the automatic timing system is to measure and terminate the exposure when sufficient radiation has reached the film to produce the desired optical density.

There are two types of automatic exposure timers:

- Timers that use a photocell or a photomultiplier tube. These timers are true phototimers because they are based on the principle of fluorescence.
- Timers that use an ionization chamber. These timers are called ionization timers because they are based on the principle of gas ionization.

The essential features of automatic timers is described in the next section. It is important to note that current state-of-the-art automatic timers use ionization chambers.

AUTOMATIC EXPOSURE CONTROL

An automatic exposure timer produces film quality with consistent optical density, regardless of the patient size, by compensating for patient thickness and radiation attenuation.

Two types of automatic systems were mentioned earlier: the phototimer and the ionization chamber.

- When automatic timers are installed, they are calibrated using a phantom. Several films of the phantom are taken with a wide range of optical densities and shown to the radiologist, who ultimately selects the range of densities to suit his or her viewing needs. This is occasionally referred to as a reference exposure level.
- The reference exposure level must also be capable of being adjusted to match the sensitivity or speed of the image receptor.

- The reference exposure level can also be adjusted using a density selector under the control of the technologist.

Phototimers

A phototimer circuit consists of a detector (a photomultiplier [PM] tube), an electronic timer circuit, density selector, and a back-up timer. The system functions as follows:

- Radiation passing through the patient falls on the detector, a fluorescent screen that is coupled to a PM tube.
- The fluorescent screen emits light that falls on the PM tube and emits electrons in direct proportion to the amount of light photons on the tube.
- The current from the PM tube is used to charge the capacitor in the electronic timer circuit.
- The switch in the electronic timer circuit opens, terminating the exposure once the desired film density is achieved.
- The charge on the capacitor determines the proper film density (that has been selected by the radiologist) on installation of the timer.

Density selection and back-up timing are described later in this chapter.

Ionization Timers

An ionization timer is the current automatic exposure control system used in radiographic imaging systems. The main component of this timer is an ionization chamber, which is a flat, parallel plate consisting of a volume of air between two metal electrodes. This volume of air is called a measuring field or a detector field (ionization detectors). Three detector fields are common (Figure 6-1). Additional major components include the AEC electronics, density control, and a back-up timer.

The system functions as follows:

- The ionization chamber measures the radiation transmitted through the patient.
- The radiation is converted into a current that is proportional to the intensity of radiation falling on the chamber. This current is used to charge the capacitor in the electronic timer circuit (AEC electronics) to a preselected value (a reference voltage). The timer switch opens

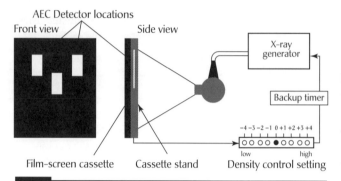

Figure 6-1 The major components of an automatic exposure control system using ionization detectors. See text for further explanation. *(From Bushberg JT, Seibert JA, Leidholdt EMJ, Boone JM, eds. The essential physics of medical imaging. Baltimore: Williams & Wilkins, 1994. Reproduced with permission.)*

(terminating the exposure) once the reference value is reached.

- When using this timer, it is vital that the anatomic part be positioned exactly over the appropriate measuring field or fields. Failure to do so will result in film with improper density.

Density Control

The technologist can select the density of a film by using the density control selector located on the control panel. The film can be made lighter or darker depending on the nature of the examination.

- When a technologist changes the density setting on the density control selector, the reference value (voltage) in the AEC electronics is changed.
- The density control goes from -4 to $+4$ settings, with a zero or normal (N) setting in the middle (see Figure 6-1).
- The optical density can be changed in steps of $\pm 10\%$ to 20% from the normal density (the density selected by the radiologist when installing the unit).
- In some systems, settings of $+1$ and $+2$ will provide a 50% and a 100% increase in mAs respectively. Settings of

−1 and −2 will provide a 25% and 50% decrease in mAs, respectively. Other systems may be programmed to provide different mAs values.

Back-Up Timer

All automatic exposure control systems are equipped with a back-up timer.

- The purpose of a back-up timer is to ensure patient safety by terminating the exposure after a preselected time (back-up time) or preselected mAs (back-up mAs) in the event of an electrical failure.
- The automatic timer can perform optimally within certain time limits, the upper time limit (back-up time) and the lower time limit (minimum response time).
- The back-up timer should be set to an exposure time that is longer (greater) than the actual or expected exposure time.
- When the back-up time is less than the actual exposure time, the exposure will terminate prematurely, and the result is an underexposed film (the film is lighter than the normal density setting).

PRACTICAL CONSIDERATIONS

The following must be considered when using exposure timers:

- For manual timers, exposure times must be selected on the basis of the technique charts established by the department. These charts list the kVp, mA, exposure time, source-to-image receptor distance (SID), and the type of image receptor that should be used for a given examination. A technologist must never guess these technique factors.
- When using automatic exposure timers on systems that allow the technologist to select any one of the kVp, mA, focal spot size, and collimation (these are referred to as partially automated systems), the following considerations are important:
  - ❑ Proper selection of the kVp. Selecting a low kVp results in poor films of varying densities. For example, barium examinations require the use of high kVp values.

❑ Altering the kVp and not the density setting can change the contrast of the image.

❑ The collimator must be adjusted to cover the entire detector field used for the examination.

❑ The anatomic region (called the dominant) must be properly positioned and aligned over the appropriate detector measuring field.

■ For fully automated systems, all technique parameters are selected automatically, when the part (anatomy) to be imaged is selected on the control panel by the technologist. These systems are called anatomically programmed radiographic (APR) systems, and they allow the technologist more time to position the patient accurately over the detector measuring field.

Advantages of Automatic Exposure Control

All modern radiographic imaging systems, including fluoroscopic systems, are equipped with automatic exposure control circuitry. These timers:

■ Provide radiographs of consistent density regardless of the size and thickness of the patient.

■ Are accurate most of the time, thus they eliminate the need for repeats resulting from exposure errors. This characteristic reduces the dose to the patient.

■ Provide more patient throughput because exposures are nearly always correct.

■ Provide automatic compensation for exposures when the SID changes.

■ Can be applied to a variety of examinations including mammography, tomography, and mobile radiography.

Quality Control for Exposure Timers

The accuracy of the exposure timer can be checked using a set of quality control (QC) tests. It is not within the scope of this chapter to describe these tests; they are discussed further in Chapter 10. The QC tests include:

■ *Spinning top test.* This test uses a spinning top to test the accuracy of exposure timers for single-phase generators.

- Synchronous spinning top for testing the accuracy of the exposure timer for three-phase and high-frequency generators.
- The use of other sophisticated test instruments such as ionization chambers and photodiode devices.
- QC test for automatic exposure timers should also be performed as part of a regular QC program for the department.
- Tolerance limit or acceptance criterion for exposure timer accuracy is ±5% for exposure times above 10 ms; ±20% can be tolerated for 10 ms or less (Bushong, 2001).
- Accurate automatic exposure timers should produce constant film density when objects of varying sizes are imaged at different kVp settings.

EXPOSURE TIME AND RADIATION PROTECTION

One of the guiding triads of radiation protection deals with the concepts of time, shielding, and distance. It is not within the scope of this chapter to describe these concepts and how they influence radiation dose. However, the technologist must note that:

- Exposure is directly proportional to time. Increasing the exposure time increases the dose; that is, doubling the exposure time increases the dose by a factor of two.
- Exposure time should always be kept as short as possible to minimize dose to the patient in both radiography and fluoroscopic procedures.

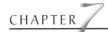
Equipment for Controlling Scattered Radiation

Chapter at a glance

When radiation interacts with the patient, part of the beam is absorbed, a portion is transmitted through the patient to strike the image receptor, and part of it is scattered through various angles. The scattered radiation transmitted through the patient reaches the film and degrades image quality. Specifically, scattered radiation reduces image contrast.

This chapter describes various equipment and methods used to improve image contrast by reducing the amount of scattered radiation reaching the film. Additionally, the factors affecting the production of scattered radiation are reviewed.

An understanding of these topics will guide the technologist in making informed decisions regarding the trade-off between image quality and radiation dose. The techniques for improving image contrast will also affect exposure technique factors that have an influence on patient dose.

Origin of Scattered Radiation

Scattered radiation has its origin in the Compton scattering process (or the Compton effect). There are five ways that x-rays can interact with matter: classical scattering, Compton scattering, photoelectric effect, pair production, and photo disintegration. In diagnostic radiology, two of these interactions predominate: Compton scattering and the photoelectric effect. Of these two, the Compton effect explains the origin of scattered radiation.

- Compton scattering involves the interaction between an incident photon and outer shell electrons that are loosely bound. The interaction results in the following:
  - Scattered photons (with less energy than the incident photons) that leave the atom in different directions. Photons that are scattered in a forward direction (direction of the primary beam) reach the film. The scattered radiation that reaches the film reduces image contrast.
  - Positive atomic ions, since incident photons remove electrons from the atom (ionization). These electrons are called Compton electrons.
- The probability of Compton scattering is inversely proportional to the incident photon energy. As the energy (kilovolts peak [kVp]) increases, the probability of Compton scattering decreases.
- Compton interaction produces radiation scattered in all directions in the x-ray room, which creates a hazard for occupational exposure.

❑ In radiography, this hazard is not serious for technologists since they should always be in the shielded control booth during exposures.

❑ In fluoroscopy, the hazard is considered serious because workers are present in the room during the procedure. In this case, protective shielding is mandatory.

FACTORS AFFECTING THE AMOUNT OF SCATTER PRODUCTION

The factors affecting the amount of scattered radiation produced in the patient are the energy of the radiation beam expressed in kVp, radiation field size, and patient thickness.

Radiation Field Size

The radiation field size is affected by the collimator, which can be adjusted manually or automatically to limit or restrict the beam to the anatomic area of interest. As the field size (square inches) increases, the relative intensity of scatter radiation increases.

Patient Thickness

The thickness of the irradiated tissue affects the amount of scattered radiation produced in the patient. Thicker body parts will produce more scattered radiation compared with thinner body parts, because a larger volume of tissue is irradiated.

kVp

As the kVp is increased, image contrast decreases. A film taken with a high kVp technique appears to have less contrast than one taken with a low-kVp technique.

■ As the kVp increases, the relative number of Compton interactions (as opposed to photoelectric interactions) increases. More radiation is scattered in a forward direction and reaches the film to destroy image contrast.

■ For example, at 90 kVp, the percentage photoelectric and Compton interactions are 38% and 59%, respectively; the interaction is 18% and 83%, respectively, for a 120 kVp beam. Additionally, the percentage transmission through 10 cm of tissue at 120 kVp is 9% compared with 3% at 90 kVp (Bushong, 2001).

SOURCES OF SCATTERED RADIATION

The main source of scattered radiation in radiography and fluoroscopy is the patient. Other sources of scatter are the x-ray tube housing, the collimator, the x-ray table, the image receptor, and the floor. To reduce occupational exposure, it is mandatory to remain as far away as possible from these sources of scatter.

IMPROVING CONTRAST: ANTISCATTER TECHNIQUES

An antiscatter technique is one that is intended to reduce the amount of scattered radiation reaching the film. The purpose of an antiscatter technique is to improve image contrast by reducing the amount of scattered radiation reaching the image receptor.

Antiscatter techniques include low-kVp techniques, compression, field size limitation, the air-gap technique, scattered radiation grid technique, and the use of scanning slit assemblies. The essentials of the first four are reviewed here; details of the antiscatter grid and scanning slits are outlined in a separate section.

Low kVp Technique

The kVp determines the beam energy or the penetrating power of the photons. To improve image contrast from scatter degradation:

- Choose a low-kVp technique since photoelectric effect predominates. It is important to realize, however, that patient dose increases as the kVp decreases.
- The technologist must note that there is a trade-off between image contrast and patient dose. As the kVp increases, scatter increases (the scattered photons have a higher energy and are therefore more penetrating), thus degrading image contrast (Figure 7-1).

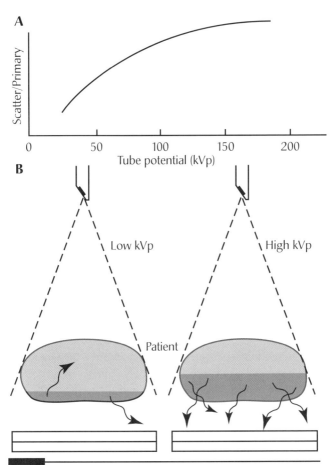

Figure 7-1 Scatter radiation degradation of image contrast tends to increase with photon energy. *A,* Scatter-to-primary ratio as a function of kVp. *B,* Image degrading scatter comes largely from the part of the patient's anatomy that lies closest to the image receptor. As photon energy increases, there is an increase in the volume of tissue in which are produced scattered photons that can escape the body. Also, scatter photons are more likely to come off in a more forward direction, toward the image receptor. *(From Wolbarst AB. Physics of radiology. Norwalk, CT: Appleton and Lange, 1993. Used with permission.)*

Field Size Limitation: Collimation

The collimator or any other beam restrictor controls the size of the x-ray beam directed to the patient and the image receptor.

- Beam restricting devices include cones, cylinders, variable-aperture collimators, diaphragms, and extension cylinders.
- Among these devices, the variable-aperture collimator is the most popular because it can shape the field size by moving pairs of lead leaves to produce square or rectangular field sizes. This action is referred to as collimation.
- Positive beam limitation (PBL) refers to automatic field collimation. A PBL system ensures that the primary beam is collimated automatically to the size of the image receptor placed in the Bucky tray.

To improve image contrast from scatter degradation influenced by the x-ray beam field size:

- Use the smallest possible field size for the examination. That is, collimate the beam to the size of the image receptor or smaller.
- The International Commission on Radiological Protection (ICRP) states that, in terms of the factors affecting the dose to the patient, the most significant is limiting the x-ray field size to the anatomic area of interest.
- Collimation reduces the genetically significant dose (GSD = the population gonadal dose) by 65%.
- Collimator filtration. Remember that the purpose of filtration is to protect the patient by removing the low-energy photons from the x-ray beam, since these photons do not play a role in image formation.
  - ❏ The total permanent filtration of the x-ray beam includes inherent, added, and collimator filtration.
  - ❏ Collimator filtration is a result of the mirror and the plastic beam definer (exit portal) of the collimator. This filtration is approximately 1.0 mm aluminum equivalent.

Compression Technique

The compression technique is often used in examinations to decrease patient thickness. A compression device such as a compression band can be used to compress the tissue and reduce the overall thickness of the patient. With a reduction in the thickness of the tissue, there is also a reduction in the amount of scattered radiation reaching the film, resulting in an improvement of image contrast.

Air-Gap Technique

This technique (also referred to as *air filtration*) uses a gap (approximately 10 to 15 cm) between the patient and the image receptor, large enough to prevent scattered radiation from the patient from reaching the film. Because scattered rays are more divergent than primary rays, they fall out of the gap and never reach the image receptor. In this way, film contrast is improved.

Because the object is not close to the image receptor, the air-gap technique will result in image magnification. To solve this problem:

- A longer source-to-image receptor distance (SID) is used. Based on the geometry of a long SID beam, the rays at the image receptor are almost parallel, thereby reducing magnification.

- Because of the increased SID, technique factors (milli-amperage and time in seconds [mAs]) should be increased to maintain the same film density.

- Although there is an increase in the mAs, the dose to the patient remains the same. For example, two chest examinations performed at 180 cm and 300 cm deliver the same 10 mR to the patient when 120 kVp and 2 mAs and when 120 kVp and 6.5 mAs are used respectively (Bushong, 2001).

- "The air-gap technique is not effective with high-kVp radiography because in high-kVp radiography the direction of the scattered rays is toward the film. At tube potentials below approximately 90 kVp, the scattered x-rays are directed more to the side and therefore have a higher probability of being scattered away from the film. Nevertheless, in some departments, 120 to 140 kVp air-gap chest radiography is used with good results" (Bushong, 2001).

Scattered Radiation Grids

Apart from the antiscatter techniques described thus far, another widely used approach to improve image contrast is to use an antiscatter device called a radiographic grid.

The grid is made up of a series of extremely thin strips of lead alternating with extremely thin strips of radiolucent material, such as aluminum or plastic fiber. The grid is placed between the patient and the image receptor to improve image contrast by absorbing radiation scattered by the patient.

Because the grid is an important and popular tool for improving image contrast, it is reviewed in detail in the next section.

Antiscatter Grids: Design and Performance

The design and performance characteristics of the grid that are of significance to the technologist in terms of image quality and dose to the patient include:

- Grid design features
- Grid clean-up efficiency
- Types of grids
- Performance characteristics, such as the grid ratio, grid frequency, contrast improvement factor, Bucky factor, selectivity, and patient dose
- Grid cutoff
- High strip-density grids
- Clinical selection of grids
- Limitations of antiscatter grids

Grid Design

A grid is made up of thin strips of radiopaque material alternating with thin strips of radiolucent material.

- The radiopaque material is also called the *grid material* and is usually made of lead. These lead strips or grid strips are approximately 50 μm thick.
- The grid material must have high absorption characteristics, high density, and a high atomic number. Although several materials (gold, tungsten) fulfill these requirements, lead is used since its atomic number is 82 and its density is 11.35 gm/cm^3. These two properties make lead an effective absorber of scattered radiation. Lead is also inexpensive and can be easily shaped into thin strips.

■ The radiolucent material or *interspace material* supports the lead strips and holds them firmly and securely in place. The thickness of each interspace strip is approximately 350 μm. Interspace materials can be aluminum or plastic fiber. The atomic number for aluminum is higher than it is for plastic fiber and absorbs more scattered rays than plastic fiber.

❑ Patient dose may be increased by approximately 20% with aluminum at low-kVp techniques.

❑ Aluminum is non-hygroscopic (will not absorb moisture) and will not warp as plastic fiber material.

❑ The height of the lead strips (thus the grid) is approximately 3 mm.

❑ The entire assembly of lead strips and interspace strips is encased in aluminum to provide mechanical rigidity and to keep moisture out of the assembly.

Grid Clean-Up Efficiency

The alternating strips of lead and interspace material are arranged to absorb scattered rays that are more oblique than the primary rays.

■ This removal of scattered radiation is referred to as *clean-up efficiency*.

■ A properly designed grid can remove 80% to 90% of scattered radiation thus providing a marked improvement of image contrast.

■ The percentage absorption of radiation incident on a grid can be calculated as follows:

$$\% \text{ absorption} = \frac{\text{grid strip thickness}}{\text{interspace strip thickness} + \text{grid strip thickness}} \times 100$$

Types of Grids

There are at least three types of grids that are based on the arrangement of their radiopaque and radiolucent alternating strips: the linear parallel grid, the focused grid, and the crossed grid.

■ In the linear parallel grid, all strips are parallel to each other. A major problem with the use of this grid is called grid cut-off, in which some of the primary radiation does not reach the image receptor but are attenuated by the lead strips. This problem occurs particularly with a short SID or with a large image receptor, such as a 14- × 17-inch cassette.

❏ The grid cut-off formula is given by:

$$\text{Distance to cut-off} = \frac{\text{SID}}{\text{grid ratio}}$$

❏ Grid cut-off causes a variation in optical density across the film. This variation depends on not only the SID, but also on how the primary beam is centered to the grid's central axis (the line in the middle of the grid that is parallel to the grid strips).

❏ A linear grid removes radiation scattered in only one direction, on the long axis of the grid.

■ In a *crossed grid*, two linear grids are stacked one on top of the other thus their grid strips form a crosshatch design. That is, their strips are oriented perpendicular to each other.

❏ A cross grid can now absorb radiation scattered in two directions and has a higher clean-up efficiency than a linear grid.

❏ Crossed grids are not commonly used because they require a good deal of precision during positioning of the grid and when angled techniques are important.

■ In a *focused grid*, the grid and interspace strips are divergent (rather than being parallel to each other), thus that they coincide with the divergent rays of the primary beam at the image receptor.

❏ The focused grid must be used at a specified focal distance. However, some degree of latitude is allowed. For example, a focused grid, intended to be used at 100 cm SID, can also be used at an SID ranging from 90 to 110 cm. This aspect makes it suitable for use in the Bucky.

■ If the described grids are used in a stationary position during the exposure, then grid lines appear on the film as thin, white lines. These lines can be removed by moving the grid during the exposure.

- The *Potter-Bucky diaphragm* or Bucky consists of a focused grid with an electronic circuit for moving the grid and a tray for holding the film cassette. The Bucky is intended to remove grid lines by moving the grid systematically during the exposure.

Grid lines may still appear when the Bucky is in use. The common cause for this is a phenomenon referred to as the *stroboscopic effect,* which occurs when the x-ray pulses produced by the generator are not synchronized with the motion of the grid.

Performance Characteristics

The performance characteristics of a grid explain how the grid removes scattered radiation and the consequences of this removal on image quality and radiation dose. These characteristics include the grid ratio, the grid frequency, the contrast improvement factor, the Bucky factor, and the selectivity.

- The *grid ratio* is one of the most significant grid characteristics and is relevant to the daily activities of the technologist. The grid ratio is given by the following relationship:

$$\text{grid ratio} = \frac{\text{ratio of the height of grid strip}}{\text{thickness of the interspace material}}$$

  - ❏ Grid ratios can range from 5:1 to 16:1.
  - ❏ Common grid ratios are 8:1, 10:1, and 12:1.
  - ❏ A higher grid ratio equals better clean-up efficiency of the grid and better image contrast. Whereas, this is 85% for a 5:1 grid, it is 97% for a 16:1 grid.
  - ❏ When the grid ratio is higher, the dose to the patient is greater.
  - ❏ High-ratio grids are best suited for examinations requiring high kVp techniques.
- The *grid frequency,* also called the strip density, is the number of grid strips (or lines) per centimeter.
  - ❏ As the grid frequency increases, the dose to the patient increases.
  - ❏ Grid frequencies range from 25 to 45 lines/cm.
  - ❏ As the grid frequency increases, the interspace material must be thinner, and the grid ratio becomes higher.

❑ High strip density (HSD) grids are now available to reduce the line pattern interference produced by conventional low strip density (LSD) grids. The grid frequency for HSD grids is about 57 lines/cm.

■ The *contrast improvement factor* (k), as opposed to the grid ratio, is a measure of how much improvement in contrast is achieved when using a grid, which can be calculated using the following relationship:

$$k = \frac{\text{image contrast with a grid}}{\text{image contrast without a grid}}$$

❑ When k = 1, there is no contrast improvement.
❑ In general, k can range from 1.5 to 2.5 for popular grids.
❑ "The contrast improvement factor is usually measured at 100 kVp, but it should be realized that k is a complex function of the x-ray emission spectrum, the patient thickness, and the area irradiated. Generally, the contrast improvement factor is higher for high-ratio grids. Other factors, such as lead content, also influence this measure of grid performance" (Bushong, 2001).

■ The *Bucky factor* (BF), often called the *grid factor*, is a performance characteristic that indicates the increase of the dose to the patient when a grid is used. The BF is a ratio of the exposure with a grid to the exposure without a grid. Values for BF can range from 2 to 6 (1 = no grid) depending on the grid ratio and the kVp.
❑ The BF increases with increasing kVp and increasing grid ratio. For example, the BF for a 5:1 grid is 2, and a 12:1 grid is 3.5 at 70 kVp. However, the BF is 3 for a 5:1 grid and 5 for a 12:1 grid at 120 kVp (Bushong, 2001).
❑ A higher BF means increased patient dose. Because the increase in BF from a 12:1 to a 16:1 is not significant, a 12:1 ratio grid is preferable for most clinical examinations.

■ The *selectivity* of a grid is a ratio of the transmitted primary radiation to the transmitted scattered rays through the grid. Selectivity takes into account not only the grid ratio, but also the amount of lead used to make the grid strips.

❑ Increasing the amount of lead increases the selectivity.

❑ With an increase in the selectivity, the grid performance (removal of scattered radiation) is improved.

Clinical Use of Grids

Grids are used in two situations in Radiology. They are part of the Bucky mechanism in the department, thus they are of the moving type. They are also used as stationary grids in mobile and operating room radiography.

■ Always use an HSD grid to reduce the visual appearance of grid lines when conducting mobile radiography.

■ Always use a grid when the anatomic part is thicker than 12 cm or techniques that use greater than 70 kVp to improve image contrast.

■ *Grid cut-off problems* are frequently encountered with the use of stationary focused grids. Common problems include:

❑ *Lateral decentering:* A condition in which the central ray of the primary beam is not centered to the middle of the grid. This condition will result in a loss of density over the entire film, since primary radiation is absorbed uniformly by all grid strips.

❑ *Off-focus error:* A condition in which the grid is used at the incorrect SID. For closer than the specified SID, there is a loss in density at the periphery of the film. For greater than the specified SID, the effect is the same as mentioned but there is a less pronounced loss in density at the periphery compared with the middle of the film.

❑ *Upside-down error:* A condition in which the grid has been turned upside-down. That is, the tube side of the grid is not facing the tube. In this case, the grid strips at the periphery of the grid absorb the primary oblique rays, although some primary rays pass through the center of the grid. This condition has the effect of producing a narrow strip of density in the middle of the film.

❑ *Lateral decentering:* A condition in which the incorrect focusing distance with either greater or smaller focusing distance. For both, the density effect is the same. That is, there is a loss of density on one side of the film compared with the other side, which is considerably darker.

■ For thicker anatomic parts, higher ratio grids will produce better image quality.

■ High-kVp techniques require the use of higher ratio grids. For example, an 8:1 linear grid can best be used with a kVp level of up to 100; a 12:1 linear grid can be used with a level above 110 kVp.

■ When going from nongrid to grid applications, changes in radiographic exposure technique factors (mAs and kVp) are required. The grid ratios of 5:1, 8:1, 12:1, and 16:1 require an mAs increase 2, 4, 5, and 6 times, respectively, from a non-grid technique. Similarly, these same ratios require a kVp increase of 8 to 10, 13 to 15, 20 to 25, and 30 to 40, respectively, from a non-grid technique (Bushong, 2001).

Patient Dose Considerations

The radiation dose to the patient always increases whenever a grid is used.

■ Compared with a stationary grid, a moving grid requires approximately a 15% increase in the amount of radiation required for the examination.

■ High-ratio grids require more radiation exposure, increasing the dose to the patient. For example, the entrance dose for an 8:1 grid is 325 mrad, compared with 425 mrad for a 12:1 grid at 70 kVp with a 200-speed image receptor (Bushong, 2001).

■ When the clinical examination requires high kVp techniques, high-ratio grids provide the best image quality.

■ High-kVp techniques result in a smaller dose to the patient because most of the radiation is transmitted through the patient to get to the image receptor. For example, the entrance dose at 70 kVp, 90 kVp, and 110 kVp, using a 12:1 ratio grid and a 200-speed image receptor system, is 425 mrad, 395 mrad, and 290 mrad, respectively.

- High-ratio grids and high kVp techniques will produce the same image quality as do low-ratio grids and low-kVp techniques, with less radiation dose to the patient.

Scanning Slit Assemblies

A scanning slit assembly is yet another antiscatter device used to improve image contrast by removal of scattered radiation.

Limitations of Antiscatter Grids

The conventional antiscatter grid has several shortcomings. The grid:

- Does not transmit the primary beam efficiently because of absorption of the beam by the grid strips, the interspace material, and the grid casing material.
- Increases the dose to the patient.

Scanning Slit Assemblies

These assemblies have been developed as early as 1902 and research continues to examine their use as effective antiscatter devices. The goal of this scanning technique is to overcome the problems imposed by grids.

- A scanning slit assembly consists of two sets of slits (long and narrow apertures cut into a thin metal plate); a fore slit (placed before the patient) that serves to define the primary beam, and an aft slit. The aft slit is placed after the patient to prevent scatter from reaching the image receptor.
- When used during an examination, the two slits travel in the same direction at the same time to scan the anatomic area being imaged.
- Scanning slit assemblies provide significant improvement in image contrast compared with conventional grids for the same patient exposure.

These assemblies provide a practical alternative to the antiscatter grid. They provide an efficient means of improving image contrast by preventing scattered radiation from reaching the film.

CHAPTER 8

Fluoroscopic Imaging Systems

Chapter at a glance

Whereas radiographic imaging systems produce static or stationary images of the patient, fluoroscopy allows the radiologist to observe dynamic or moving images on a television monitor for the purpose of studying both structure and function of organ systems.

During a fluoroscopic examination the radiologist and technologist must work together to accomplish the goal of providing excellent patient care while producing optimal image quality with as low a radiation dose as possible. The role of the technologist is vital to the success of a fluoroscopic examination. It is therefore essential that all technologists have a firm grasp of the major components and principles of fluoroscopic imaging systems. This understanding can only improve the speed and quality of the examination, and especially, guide the technologist in minimizing the dose to both the patients and the personnel working in fluoroscopy.

The purpose of this chapter is to outline three elements of a fluoroscopic examination, and identify and describe the major components of a conventional fluoroscopic imaging system. These include image intensification, x-ray television, and spot-film recording techniques. Finally, the chapter outlines the components and operation of digital fluoroscopy.

Elements of a Fluoroscopic Examination

A fluoroscopic examination includes at least three essential elements:

- **Fluoroscopy:** This process displays images in real-time on a television monitor, which requires continuous x-ray production. This part of the examination is generally carried out by the radiologist using fluoroscopic exposure technique factors.
- **Fluorography:** This process records images from the image-intensifier tube that are displayed on the television monitor. This procedure is usually carried out by the radiologist using fluoroscopic exposure technique factors.
- **Radiography:** Two techniques are used during a fluoroscopic examination:
  - ❏ *Spot-film radiography* records images by radiographic means using the *cassette-loaded spot-film device.* This

procedure is usually carried out by the radiologist. When an image of this nature is recorded, the fluoroscopic imaging system must switch from fluoroscopic exposure factors to radiographic exposure factors and back to fluoroscopic factors.

❑ *"Overhead" radiography* records images on large-format films in the Bucky using radiographic exposure technique factors. This part of the examination is carried out by the technologist after the radiologist has completed fluoroscopy.

CONVENTIONAL FLUOROSCOPY: EQUIPMENT COMPONENTS

The major equipment components of a conventional fluoroscopic imaging system include an x-ray tube for fluoroscopy and radiography, a Bucky for "overhead" radiography, a cassette-loaded spot-film device, an image intensifier tube, an optical image distributor or a fiber optical system, a closed-circuit television system, and a photo-spot film camera (Figure 8-1). (The cassette-loaded spot-film device, which is located between the patient and the image intensifier tube, is not shown in Figure 8-1.)

X-Ray Tube

The x-ray tube used in fluoroscopy must be capable of producing x-rays continuously to allow for real-time display of images. Some fluoroscopic imaging systems use x-rays produced in short bursts (pulsed fluoroscopy) rather than continuously. In this case, the x-ray tube is a grid-controlled tube. Systems that can produce pulses of less than 10 pulses per second can reduce the patient exposure by as much as 90% compared with nonpulsed systems. These tubes must be capable of providing exposure technique factors for both the fluoroscopic and the radiographic portions of the examination.

■ Fluoroscopic factors are generally low milliamperes (mA) and high kilovolts peak (kVp) with a range of 1 to 3 mA and 65 to 120 kVp, depending on the nature of the examination.

■ Radiographic factors are required when the radiologist records an image using the cassette-loaded spot-film

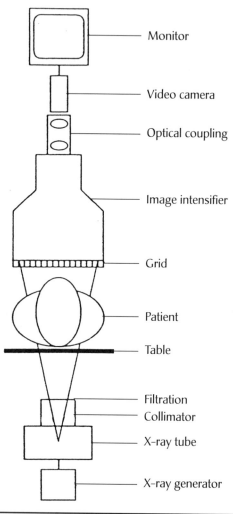

Figure 8-1 The major components of a fluoroscopic imaging system. Reproduced by permission *(From Schueller BA. General overview of fluoroscopic imaging.* Radiographics *2000;20:1115–1126.)*

device. In this case, the machine switches from the fluoroscopic mode to radiographic mode, and the tube current is switched to higher mA values.

Cassette-Loaded Spot-Film Device

Some fluoroscopic imaging systems, also known as under-
couch systems (the x-ray tube is located under the x-ray table,
with the image intensifier tube positioned above the table) use
a spot-film device to record by radiographic means the fluoroscopic image being seen on the monitor.

- The technologist loads and unloads the spot-film device
  with the appropriate sized film as required by the
  radiologist.
- Because the image intensifier tube is attached to the
  spot-film device, the radiologist moves it to scan and
  examine the anatomy under investigation.
- The radiologist can record images of varying formats on
  the film by collimating the beam during the examination.
- Among the image-recording modes used in fluoroscopy,
  the cassette-loaded spot-film device produces the best
  image quality but requires the highest radiation dose.
- The use of the cassette-loaded spot-film device tends to
  increase the length of time necessary for the fluoroscopic portion of the examination. This condition is attributed to the time taken to load and unload the device.
  Using photo-spot camera recording techniques can
  solve this problem.

Image Intensifier Tube

The *image intensifier* tube is a special electronic tube that overcomes the problems of a conventional fluoroscopic screen. For
this reason, it is described in detail in the next section.

The purpose of the image intensifier tube is to convert x-ray
photons from the patient to light photons. The image is brighter
than the conventional fluoroscopic screen image. This bright
image cannot be viewed directly by the observer thus it must be
transmitted for suitable viewing using a closed-circuit television
system.

Optical Image Distributor-Fiber Optics

The *image distributor* is coupled with the output screen of the image intensifier tube and consists of a series of lenses and a beam-splitting mirror.

- The purpose of the image distributor is to distribute the total light output from the output screen of the intensifier tube between the television camera tube, or *charge-coupled device* (CCD), and the photo-spot film camera.

- 10% of the light travels to the television camera or CCD and 90% reaches the photo-spot film camera.

- In some systems (portable fluoroscopic units) fiber optics is used to couple the image intensifier tube with the television camera tube or CCD. Fiber optics has the advantage of compactness, and it allows for easy handling of the image intensifier.

Closed-Circuit Television

A *closed-circuit television* system for fluoroscopic imaging consists of a television camera tube (or a CCD unit), a coaxial cable, a signal electronics unit, and a television picture tube or a television monitor, as it is often called.

- The *television camera* tube is a photo-electronic tube that converts visual information; that is, the light from the output screen of the image intensifier tube is converted into an electronic signal. This signal is called the video signal.

- The CCD has replaced the television camera tube in modern fluoroscopic imaging systems. This solid-state electronic device is also used in personal video cameras. The CCD captures the light from the image intensifier output screen and converts it into a video signal.

- The *coaxial cable* connects the television camera tube/CCD to the television monitor via the signal electronics unit, which conducts the output video signal to the monitor. The conductor (wire) runs down the center of the cable, which has a protective, grounded metal sheath surrounding it.

- The *television monitor* or *picture tube* converts the output video signal (electrical signal) received from the television camera tube-CCD into a visual image or the fluoroscopic image.

Photo-Spot Camera

Photo-spot cameras are used to record fluoroscopic images from the output screen of the intensifier tube.

- The photo-spot camera uses variable film sizes ranging from 90 to 105 mm. However, the 105 mm format has become popular and is now used in fluoroscopic systems. This small film format is occasionally perceived as a disadvantage.

- The radiologist operates the photo-spot camera to record fluoroscopic images viewed on the television monitor. Photo-spot image recording is preferred over cassette-loaded spot-film recording because:

  ❏ Less radiation dose is required (fluoroscopic exposure technique factors, low mA, and high kVp are used) compared with cassette-loaded spot-film recording. The image quality, however, is not as good as the large format cassette-loaded film images. A resolution of four line pairs per millimeter is possible with photo-spot film cameras. The radiation dose is approximately 2 to 3 times less than that of cassette-loaded film imaging.

  ❏ The fluoroscopic imaging portion of the examination can be completed faster than when cassette-loaded spot-films are used because the interruption resulting from loading and unloading the spot-film device by the technologists is eliminated.

  ❏ There is less heat loading on the x-ray tube because low-mA and high-kVp techniques are used to record images.

  ❏ Patient motion artifacts are reduced because short exposure times (approximately 50 ms) are used.

X-Ray Image Intensifier Tube

Before the advent of the image intensifier tube, radiologists performed fluoroscopy by direct observation of images on a *fluorescent screen*. The screen was made of *zinc cadmium sulfide* (ZnCdS) and fluoresced yellow-green when struck by x-rays. *Conventional fluoroscopy* had to be performed in the dark because the image lacked detail, brightness, and contrast. The ability to perceive detail was restricted by geometric factors, rod vision, and the low levels of brightness characteristic of the screen.

- The image intensifier tube was developed to solve the problems imposed by the conventional fluorescent screen, through a process referred to as image intensification.

- *X-ray image intensification* is the brightening of the conventional fluoroscopic image using the image intensifier tube.

- The major components of an x-ray image intensifier tube include an input phosphor, photo cathode, electrostatic focusing lenses, and an output phosphor (Figure 8-2). These components are housed in an evacuated glass envelope.

Input Phosphor

The *input phosphor* is a fluorescent screen that absorbs and converts x-ray photons received from the patient into light photons.

- The phosphor material used in state-of-the-art image intensifiers is *cesium iodide* (CsI) as opposed to zinc cadmium sulfide (ZnCdS), characteristic of first- and second-generation intensifiers.

- CsI absorbs twice as much radiation, compared with ZnCdS, thus reducing the exposure required for image formation.

- CsI crystals are packed in a needle-like fashion and are arranged in the direction in which the x-ray photons travel. This arrangement reduces the lateral dispersion of light, resulting in better spatial resolution compared with ZnCdS intensifiers.

- Input phosphor screens have diameters ranging from 13 to 30 cm, with 15 and 23 cm being the most common. Recently, large diameters (36 and 57 cm) have become available for use in imaging large anatomic regions such as the abdomen.

Photocathode

The light photons from the input phosphor strike a photocathode that emits photoelectrons in direct proportion to the amount of light photons it receives.

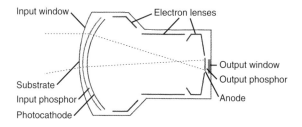

Figure 8-2 The major components of an x-ray image intensifier tube used in fluoroscopy. *(From Schueller BA. General overview of fluoroscopic imaging.* Radiographics *2000; 20:1115-1126. Used with permission.)*

- The photocathode uses a photoemissive material such as cesium antimony, which will emit 5 electrons per 100 light photons.
- Multialkali photocathodes use a combination of antimony, potassium, sodium, and cesium, which emit 3 to 5 times more electrons than cesium antimony photocathodes.

Electrostatic Focusing Lenses
The electrostatic lens system consists of a series of cylindrical electrodes (positively charged) (see Figure 8-2). The *electrostatic lenses* accelerate and focus the photoelectrons from the photocathode (since there is a potential of approximately 25 to 35 kVp between the photocathode and the anode) to strike the output phosphor at high speeds.

Output Phosphor
The purpose of the *output phosphor* is to convert the photoelectrons received from the photocathode into visible light.
- The output phosphor material is zinc cadmium sulfide deposited on the inside of an optical faceplate.
- The diameter of the output phosphor is approximately one-tenth the diameter of the input phosphor.
- The image at the output phosphor is extremely small, bright, and inverted. This image cannot be viewed directly by the radiologist. Therefore it is captured by a closed-circuit television system.

Intensifier Tube Housing

The image intensifier glass envelope is encased in a housing.

- The housing provides mechanical support for the glass envelope and shields the intensifier against magnetic fields.
- The housing also provides shielding against radiation that passes through and is scattered by the input phosphor, as well as radiation that may be produced by the high-speed electrons striking the output phosphor.

Brightness Gain

The intensifier tube is efficient at each stage of the x-ray conversion process leading to the increase in brightness at the output phosphor (Table 8-1). The brightness gain (BG) is increased in the illumination (brightness) of the fluoroscopic image formed at the output phosphor.

- BG = minification gain (MG) × flux gain (FG)

- $$MG = \left[\frac{\text{diameter of input phosphor}}{\text{diameter of output phosphor}} \right]^2$$

- $$FG = \left[\frac{\text{number of light photons emitted at the output phosphor}}{\text{number of x-ray photons at the input phosphor}} \right]$$

- The BG for image intensifiers can range from 5000 to 30,000 (Bushong, 2001).

Conversion Factor

The use of the brightness gain to measure the intensification of an image intensifier tube has been replaced by a more modern method. This method uses the conversion factor to measure the light gain at the output phosphor.

- The *conversion factor* is a ratio of the luminance (light brightness) of the output phosphor to the exposure rate (mR/min) at the input phosphor.
- *Luminance* has units of candela per square meter (cd/m^2).
- The conversion factor for image intensifiers can range from 50 to 300, corresponding to brightness gains of 5000 to 30,000 (Bushong, 2001).

TABLE 8-1	Efficiency of the X-Ray Image Intensifier	
IMAGE INTENSIFIER STAGE	EFFICIENCY	NUMBER PER INCIDENT 50–keV X-RAY
Input phosphor (x-ray absorption)	50%	0.5 Photoelectrons
Input phosphor (light generation)	15%	1875 (2 eV) Light photons
Photocathode (electron emission)	10%	187 Photoelectrons
Output phosphor (electron absorption)	90%	170 Energetic electrons
Output phosphor (light generation)	10%	170,000 Light photons

The efficiency of the x-ray image intensifier tube at each stage of the x-ray conversion process lead to an increase in brightness at the output phosphor. *(From Huda W, Slone R. Review of radiological physics. Baltimore: Williams & Wilkins, 1995. Reproduced with permission.)*

■ As the image intensifier ages, its brightness level decreases. In this case, exposures (dose) must be increased to ensure the appropriate brightness at the output phosphor.

Image Magnification

During fluoroscopy, the radiologist may use magnification to facilitate viewing and interpretation of the image on the television monitor.

■ *Magnification* is only possible with *multifield image intensifier tubes*. These include dual- and tri-field tubes that use a technique called *electron-optical magnification*. With this technique, the voltage on specific electrodes (of the electrostatic lens system) is changed to cause a wider divergence of the electron beam.

■ A dual-field intensifier can be operated in two modes. In a full-field mode, the x-ray beam falls on the full diameter of the input phosphor (25 cm for a 25 cm/17 cm, dual-mode intensifier). In the second mode, the magnification mode, the x-ray beam is collimated to fall on the central portion of the input phosphor covering a diameter of 17 cm.

■ A tri-field image intensifier tube can be operated in three modes. Typical tri-field modes are 25/17/12 and 23/15/10. The magnification modes are 17 and 12 cm, and 15 and 10 cm, respectively.

- Image quality (spatial resolution) is significantly better in the magnification mode, but at the expense of increased dose to the patient. The dose increase is approximately 2.2 times the dose when the full-field mode is used. This dose can be calculated using the ratio of the full-field diameter squared to the magnified field diameter (central portion of the input phosphor) squared. For a 25/17 intensifier the dose increase in the magnification mode (17 cm) is $25^2/17^2$ (Bushong, 2001).

Image Quality Considerations

Image intensifier image quality can be discussed in terms of spatial resolution, contrast, noise, and artifacts.

- *Spatial resolution.* Spatial resolution is the ability of the intensifier to resolve fine detail. The resolution is substantially better in the central portion of the input phosphor compared with the periphery. The resolution is 4 lp/mm in a 25 cm mode (for a CsI intensifier) and 6 lp/mm in a 10 cm mode, which means that 0.125 mm objects can be seen with 4 lp/mm compared with 0.08 mm sized objects at 6 lp/mm (Bushong, 2001).
- *Contrast.* Image intensifier contrast is defined as the ratio of the light intensity at the periphery to the light intensity at the center of the output screen. A typical contrast ratio is 20:1. Image intensification results in a loss of contrast as a result of:
  - Few photons incident on the input phosphor penetrate it, as well as the photocathode, to strike the output phosphor.
  - *Retrograde light flow* (few light photons) at the output phosphor, traveling back to the photocathode to generate additional electrons.
  - *Veiling glare* (scattering and reflection of light in the intensifier tube).
- *Noise.* The noise (quantum mottle) level of an image intensifier is usually high because low tube currents are used in fluoroscopy. To reduce the noise, more photons must strike the input screen, which can be achieved by increasing the mA. However, there will be a corresponding increase in patient dose. A CsI intensifier exhibits

less noise than a ZnCdS intensifier, since CsI has a higher quantum detection efficiency.

■ *Artifacts.* Artifacts arising in an image intensifier result from lag, vignetting, and pincushion distortion. Although lag implies continued luminescence after the x-ray beam has been turned off, vignetting is a loss of brightness at the periphery of the image. Pincushion distortion, conversely, refers to an increase in magnification of the image at the periphery resulting from "inadequate electronic focusing" (Huda and Slone, 1995). This type of distortion decreases as the diameter of the input phosphor increases and is about 3% for a 23-cm intensifier tube (Huda and Slone, 1995).

CLOSED-CIRCUIT X-RAY TELEVISION

The image at the output phosphor is too small and too bright to be viewed directly by the radiologist. This image is monitored and displayed for proper viewing by a closed circuit television system. This is sometimes referred to as *television fluoroscopy*.

The major components of a television system for fluoroscopy are a television camera tube (or a CCD unit) and the television monitor, connected by a coaxial cable.

Television Camera Tubes

A *television* (TV) *camera* is coupled with the output phosphor via the image distributor. The purpose of the TV camera is to "pick up" the image at the output phosphor and convert it into an electrical signal (output video signal). This signal is sent to the TV monitor.

Two types of camera tubes are used in fluoroscopy: the vidicon or the plumbicon, because they are smaller and not as complex as image orthicons.

■ The *vidicon* and the *plumbicon* are based on the principle of photoconductivity and differ in respect to their photoconductors. The vidicon uses antimony trisulfide and the plumbicon uses lead oxide.

■ The vidicon is simple and compact, with reduced image distortion and less noise in the signal. However, it suffers increased image lag at low levels of brightness and has reduced image contrast.

■ The plumbicon has improved image contrast and reduced image lag compared with the vidicon. However, the plumbicon is expensive and slightly larger than the vidicon. The plumbicon also produces a decrease in detail visibility.

TV camera tubes are cylindrical in shape (25 mm diameter and 15 cm long) and consists of a photoconductive target at one end and an electron gun at the other end.

The TV tube works as follows:

■ The image at the output phosphor of the intensifier tube falls on the photoconductive target plate of the TV camera tube.

■ At the same time, an electron beam produced by the electron gun scans the target plate.

■ Because the signal plate is photoconductive, it emits electrons when light (from the output phosphor) falls on it.

■ When electrons from the electron gun strike the same part of the target that emits electrons, a video signal is produced.

■ Video signal strength is proportional to the amount of light falling on the target. When the light intensity is increased, the strength of the video signal is increased. No light means that no signal will be generated.

■ The output video signal from the TV camera contains the data from the patient and is sent to the TV monitor that converts it into a visible image.

Charge-Coupled Devices

Charge-coupled devices (CCDs) have replaced TV cameras in modern fluoroscopic imaging systems because they offer significant advantages compared with TV camera tubes, including uniform resolution over the entire image and low readout noise. A visual comparison of the resolution between CCD and a TV camera tube (Figure 8-3).

The CCD array is positioned in the center of the camera head (Figure 8-4) and consists of a target matrix, which contains a large number of pixels. A matrix size of 1024 × 1024 is common. The CCD works as follows:

- The light from the output phosphor of the image intensifier tube falls on the CCD pixels. Each pixel contains a photosensitive region that produces electrons when struck by light.
- The electron charge from each pixel is read out systematically using a series of electronic registers.
- The output signal (video signal) from the CCD is sent to a camera control unit for a digital signal processing to reduce the noise.
- The CCD signals can be sent to a computer system or to a TV monitor for image display.

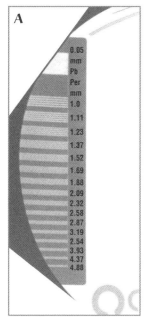

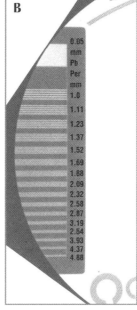

Picture of lead pattern at the edge of the X-RII field taken with a **pick-up tube camera** and a 16" X-RII (in 7" mode, x-ray dose level for radiography).

Picture of lead pattern at the edge of the X-RII field taken with the **TH 8730 CCD camera** and a 16" X-RII (in 7" mode, x-ray dose level for radiography).

Figure 8-3 *A*, A visual comparison of the resolution obtained with a TV camera tube, *B*, and a CCD camera. *(Courtesy of Thomson Tube Electronics, France.)*

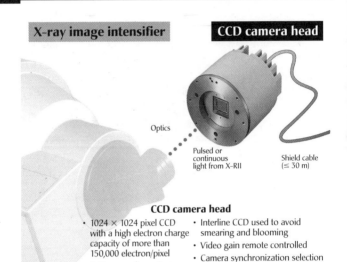

X-ray image intensifier

CCD camera head

Optics

Pulsed or
continuous
light from X-RII

Shield cable
(≤ 30 m)

CCD camera head

- 1024 × 1024 pixel CCD
with a high electron charge
capacity of more than
150,000 electron/pixel
- Active area dimensions:
13.1 × 13.1 mm

- Interline CCD used to avoid
smearing and blooming
- Video gain remote controlled
- Camera synchronization selection
- CCD blemish correction
(defective columns and pixels

Figure 8-4 The CCD camera head containing the CCD in the center. The CCD camera head is coupled with the output phosphor of the image intensifier tube via a compact integrated optical system that directs the light onto the CCD. *(Courtesy of Thomson Tubes Electronics, France.)*

Television Monitor

The output video signal from the TV camera tube-CCD unit is sent to a TV monitor. The purpose of the TV monitor is to convert an electrical signal (output video signal from the camera tube-CCD) into a visual image for display and viewing by the radiologist.

The monitor consists of a *cathode ray tube* (CRT) or picture tube, as it is sometimes called. The CRT contains an electron gun at one end and a wide fluorescent screen at the opposite end, which produces the TV image. This image is created as follows:

- The electron gun receives the output video signal from the camera tube-CCD and directs an electron beam to scan the CRT fluorescent screen.

- The TV image is made up of lines from the scanning process. On one hand, scanning can be *interlaced*, in which case, 262.5 odd lines (one field) are first scanned by the electron beam, followed by 262.5 even lines (one field). These two fields are interlaced to create one frame. The total number of lines is 525.
- Interlace scanning reduces flickering of the image.
- At a frequency of 60 Hz (60 cycles per second) 30 frames per second (60 fields per second) can be displayed for viewing. Flickering cannot be observed at this frame rate.
- Conversely, the electron beam can scan in a *progressive* fashion, during which each line is read sequentially (1, 2, 3, 4, and so on). This is important in digital fluoroscopy.

Television Image Quality Considerations

TV image quality can be discussed in terms of vertical resolution and horizontal resolution.

- *Vertical resolution* refers to the number of lines of active trace per frame. As the number of lines are increased, the vertical resolution increases. A 1000-line TV system provides twice the resolution, compared with a 525-line system. When a 23-cm image intensifier is used with a 525-line TV monitor, the spatial resolution is approximately 1 lp/mm (Huda and Slone, 1995).
- *Horizontal resolution* is generally equal to the vertical resolution and is determined by the bandwidth or bandpass of the video signal. *Bandwidth* is the frequency in Hertz (Hz) of the TV system. Specifically, bandwidth is the range of frequencies that the system can handle and refers to the number of times per second that the intensity of the electron beam can change.
- TV systems for fluoroscopy have bandwidths ranging from 4.5 MHz to approximately 20 MHz.
- As the bandwidth increases, the horizontal resolution increases.
- A 1000-line TV system has a bandwidth of approximately 20 MHz.

AUTOMATIC BRIGHTNESS CONTROL

All fluoroscopic imaging systems are equipped with a feature known as *automatic brightness control* (ABC) or *automatic dose-rate regulation* (ADR).

- The purpose of ABC is to maintain a constant brightness of the fluoroscopic image as viewed on the TV monitor since the brightness will vary resulting from changes in patient positioning and anatomic part thickness.

- ABC regulates the radiation incident on the intensifier input phosphor by automatically adjusting the mA and kVp to ensure a constant light intensity at the output phosphor.

- Automatic control of the mA and kVp can also lead to a reduction of radiation (dose-rate) when the beam moves from a thick anatomic part to a thinner region.

- ABC or ADR can be accomplished using either a sensor to detect the light from the output screen or an ionization chamber placed in front of the input phosphor of the intensifier to detect x-rays. Both systems must be connected to some feedback circuitry to the x-ray generator to control x-ray exposure technique factors.

RECORDING THE FLUOROSCOPIC IMAGE: SPOT-FILMING

The spatial resolution of a 525-line TV system is approximately 2 lp/mm compared with 5 lp/mm for the image intensifier. To capture the image intensifier resolution, spot-filming is required, using a photo-spot camera optically coupled with the output phosphor of the intensifier tube.

Current state-of-the-art spot-film imaging uses photo-spot cameras rather than the cine camera (movie camera).

The basic components of a spot-film camera include the aperture, the lens, and the film.

- The aperture determines the amount of light falling on the lens. A larger aperture will permit a greater amount of light to reach the lens.

- The lens collects the light then transfers and focuses the image onto the film. One characteristic of the lens is its focal length.

❑ The focal length is the distance (in millimeters) from the lens to the point at which the image on the film is in sharp focus.

❑ The focal length determines the size of the image on the film.

■ The sensitivity of the film must match the light output (wavelength or color) from the output phosphor. This is called *spectral matching*.

The image size and framing are also important in spot-filming.

The lens determines the image size, which is smaller than the actual film sizes used (35, 70, 90, and 105 mm). As the film size increases, dose increases. If the film size doubles, then four times the dose is required since the area of the image increases by four.

Framing is a technique used to determine the size of the image on the film. *Under framing* uses only a portion of the film to project all of the image. *Over framing*, conversely, uses the entire film. However, parts of the image are not included.

DIGITAL FLUOROSCOPY

Digital fluoroscopy is fluoroscopic imaging using a digital computer to process the output video signal from the TV camera tube or the CCD unit. Digital fluoroscopy has replaced conventional fluoroscopic imaging systems, and radiology departments are phasing out their old conventional fluoroscopic units.

A digital fluoroscopic imaging system has several imaging requirements that differ from a conventional fluoroscopic system. The components of a digital fluoroscopy unit are an x-ray tube and generator, an image intensifier tube, a TV camera tube or a CCD camera, an analog-to-digital converter, a computer system, an operator's control console, and a laser camera for recording hard copy images.

X-Ray Tube and Generator

The x-ray tube and generator provide the radiation beam required for digital fluoroscopy.

■ The x-ray tube is a high-capacity tube that produces x-rays in pulses (intermittently) as opposed to conventional tubes. Higher mA values are used.

- Three-phase or high-frequency generators are used to produce rapid pulsing of the x-ray beam (as short as 1 millisecond) to enable images to be recorded at rates that can vary from 1 per second to 10 per second.

Television Camera Tube/CCD Unit

The TV camera tube/CCD unit produces the output video signal containing image data from the output phosphor of the intensifier tube.

- The TV camera tube used in digital fluoroscopy must produce a high *signal-to-noise ratio* (low noise). Whereas the TV camera tube for use in conventional fluoroscopy has a signal-to-noise ratio of 200:1 (high noise), the TV camera tube for use in a digital unit should be about 1000:1 (Bushong, 2001). Images can be acquired at 30 per second.
- The CCD camera has extremely high sensitivity and low readout noise. Images can be acquired at 60 per second.

Analog-to-Digital Converter

The *analog-to-digital converter* (ADC) is an integral component of a digital fluoroscopy system and is positioned between the TV camera tube or CCD camera and the computer. The purpose of the ADC is to convert the output video signal (analog signal) from the TV camera or CCD camera into digital data for processing by the computer.

The ADC digitizes the output video signal by sampling it at certain time intervals. With more samples (parts of the signal) comes better accuracy of the ADC. The unit of the parts is the *bit* (binary digit). One bit can be either a "0" or a "1." An 8-bit ADC will divide the signal into 256 (2^8) numbers ranging from 0 to 255. Digital systems use 10- to 12-bit ADCs.

Computer System

The *computer* used in digital fluoroscopy is a *minicomputer* system, a midlevel computer that is more powerful than a microcomputer (single-chip microprocessor) and can perform complex calculations rapidly.

- The computer receives digital data from the ADC and performs some form of processing to produce the digital fluoroscopic image.

- This image can be stored on optical disks or displayed for viewing on a TV monitor.
- The image can also be printed on film using a laser camera.

Laser Camera

A *laser camera*—also referred to as a *laser film printer* or a *laser imager*—includes hardware and software to produce images on film.

- The *hardware* includes a *laser* that receives data from the computer and writes the image on the film. The laser may be a helium-neon laser that emits light with a wavelength of 633 nm.
- The *software* controls the hardware and ensures optimal image quality, calibration, and networking.
- *Laser films* are single-emulsion films with their sensitivities matched to the wavelength of the laser light. These films can be conventional (wet-processing) laser films or dry (self-processing) laser films.

Operator Control Console

The control console consists of a keyboard and a monitor connected to the computer.

- The keyboard allows the operator to communicate with the computer using the alphanumeric keys to enter details of the examination, including patient demographics. The keyboard also allows the operator to perform various image processing operations.
- The monitor displays processed images for viewing by the operator. Text and icons are also displayed to facilitate intuitive interaction with the system.

Digital Subtraction Angiography

Digital fluoroscopy is now used for routine fluoroscopy in examinations of the gastrointestinal tract. Another major application of digital fluoroscopy involves angiography, using a technique called *digital subtraction angiography* (DSA).

There are two methods of DSA: temporal subtraction and energy subtraction.

- *Temporal subtraction* involves subtraction of images in time. Usually a precontrast image (mask image) is obtained and postcontrast images are subtracted from it.

■ *Energy subtraction* involves subtraction of images based on the kVp they are recorded. Images are recorded based on subtraction of the energies slightly above and slightly below the K-absorption edge of the contrast material used for the examination.

The primary purpose of DSA is to demonstrate contrast differences of less than 1%, compared with conventional film-based angiography. Additionally, because DSA can show low-contrast tissues, less contrast material is required. Both venous and arterial administration of contrast medium can be used. However, venous injections are not popular because the image quality is poor resulting from a decrease in the level of contrast concentration in the arteries. Other advantages include:

■ *Image manipulation by the computer.* Windowing, image enhancement, and quantitative data analysis are possible.
■ *Images displayed on a TV monitor.* For instantaneous viewing by the radiologist, images are displayed on a TV monitor.

Fluoroscopic examinations demand a high degree of alertness and understanding of the factors influencing image quality and patient dose. The technologist and radiologist must work cooperatively as members of the fluoroscopy team to optimize the conduct of the examination.

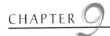

Mobile Imaging Systems

Chapter at a glance

Mobile imaging refers to *portable imaging,* either by radiography or by fluoroscopy. In this chapter, the term "portable" refers to transporting the imaging equipment to the bedside of patients who are too critically ill to travel to the main radiology department for their x-ray examination.

This chapter summarizes the fundamental principles and instrumentation of both portable radiographic and fluoroscopic units. For portable radiographic systems, the essential features of two types of units are described. For portable fluoroscopic systems, the major equipment components will be described, followed by a discussion of practical considerations when performing portable examinations.

The motivation for the study of these topics is derived from the notion that portable imaging is a routine activity for radiologic technologists. Because these patients are critically ill, are having surgery, or are traumatized, it is vital that the portable examination be conducted with the knowledge and skills to ensure optimal image quality on the first attempt. This chapter provides a small step in that direction.

RADIOGRAPHIC SYSTEMS

Portable radiographic systems can be discussed in terms of general requirements for electrical power and radiation output and in terms of the types of systems available.

General Requirements
The general requirements for portable radiographic units are:
- **Small size.** The unit should be sufficiently small and mounted on a set of wheels to allow for easy transportation and maneuverability.
- **Braking system.** The braking system allows for immobilization in situations that warrant such action.
- **Power sources.** Power outlets need to be located in all areas of the hospital. Most units require the standard 120-volt, 15-ampere power outlet. Some units do not require these outlets for x-ray production because they use large capacity, nickel-cadmium (Ni-Cd) batteries. However, because the batteries have to be recharged after use, these units must be plugged into the wall outlet for this purpose.
- **Radiation output.** Portable units have been developed to image the entire body of patients who are traumatized, who are having an operation, or who are critically ill. Because the anatomic regions vary in anatomic part thickness, one essential requirement for all portable units

is that the radiation output must be sufficient to image these regions without degradation of image quality.

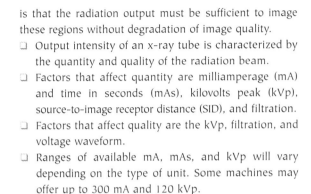

- ❏ Output intensity of an x-ray tube is characterized by the quantity and quality of the radiation beam.
- ❏ Factors that affect quantity are milliamperage (mA) and time in seconds (mAs), kilovolts peak (kVp), source-to-image receptor distance (SID), and filtration.
- ❏ Factors that affect quality are the kVp, filtration, and voltage waveform.
- ❏ Ranges of available mA, mAs, and kVp will vary depending on the type of unit. Some machines may offer up to 300 mA and 120 kVp.

- ■ *Voltage waveform.* Modern portable units have high-frequency generators that provide almost constant, ripple-free voltage to the x-ray tube. Older units have generators that provide waveforms that have a voltage ripple ranging from approximately 4% to 13%. These voltage waveforms determine the efficiency of x-ray production. High-frequency generators are more efficient than three-phase generators and therefore provide higher x-ray quantity and quality. This efficiency also allows for the use of extremely short exposure times, a technique factor that is vital when imaging patients who are critically ill.

- ■ *X-ray tubes.* Most portable x-ray machines use a rotating-anode x-ray tube. These tubes provide a higher radiation output and higher heat capacities compared with stationary-anode x-ray tubes. Higher mA values and shorter exposures are possible with rotating-anode tubes.

- ■ *Tube support.* Tube support is usually a central column consisting of a cross-arm that supports the x-ray tube. The support must provide a counterbalanced system for vertical adjustments of the tube. In addition, the tube support must provide a wide range of movements to facilitate easy positioning of the x-ray tube when imaging the patient.

- ■ *Control console.* All portable units must be provided with an operator's console that allows the technologist to turn the machine on and off, select exposure technique factors (that must be displayed as well), and make an exposure when appropriate.

- *Exposure switch.* The exposure switch on a portable x-ray unit must be of a "dead-man" type; that is, the exposure will terminate if the technologist drops dead. Actually, the switch requires continuous pressure for operation. The exposure switch must also have a coiled cord, the length of which must allow the technologist to stand at least two meters from the x-ray tube. In Canada, this length is three meters.
- *Protective apron.* All portable units should be provided with a protective lead apron for the technologist to wear during the exposure.

Capacitor-Discharge Mobile Units

The capacitor-discharge portable x-ray machine was one of the first attempts to introduce a high-powered unit capable of producing high-radiation output, using the standard 120-volt alternating current (AC) power outlet. Some hospitals may still be using these units; therefore the essentials are considered.

The basic circuitry for the generator consists of a low-voltage side and a high-voltage side. The major components of the high-voltage side are the high-voltage transformer, rectifiers, capacitors, and a grid-controlled x-ray tube.

- The capacitors are located between the rectifiers and the x-ray tube.
- The high-voltage transformer supplies high-voltage AC to the rectifiers.
- The rectifiers change the high-voltage AC into a high-voltage pulsed DC.
- The capacitors are fully charged using the output voltage from the rectifiers.
- The grid-controlled x-ray tube is used to start and stop the x-ray exposure.
  - When the grid bias is removed, the exposure commences and the capacitors discharge through the x-ray tube.
  - The exposure terminates when a bias (a few kilovolts [kV]) is placed on the grid.

The technologist must be aware of the fact that as the exposure occurs, the capacitors discharge through the x-ray tube to produce the radiation beam. The direct current (DC) voltage decreases with time. There is a 1 kVp decrease for every mAs used for the examination. For example, if an examination is done at 90 kVp at 20 mAs, then the kVp will be 70 at the end of the exposure. Additionally:

■ Higher mAs techniques will result in lower kVp values at the end of the exposure. This point is significant for large anatomic regions that require the proper kVp range for optimal penetration.

■ A decrease in the kVp results in underexposure errors and increases the dose to the patient.

■ A general rule for technique selection when using a capacitor-discharge portable machine is:
   ❑ mAs for the examination should not be greater than approximately one-third the kVp, or
   ❑ mAs should not exceed 20.

In addition to these problems, the capacitors require some time (in seconds) to become fully charged before x-ray exposure. In some units, a residual charge may remain on the tube at the termination of the exposure. Therefore to reduce the possibility of electrical shock, the unit must be discharged before it is used again.

Battery-Powered Mobile Units

To address the problems previously identified, the battery-powered mobile x-ray machine was introduced. This unit does not require a high-current wall outlet for its operation. For this reason, the battery-powered mobile x-ray machine has been referred to as the *"cordless mobile"* x-ray machine. The major components of the generator of a battery-powered mobile x-ray machine and the associated voltage waveform are shown in Figure 9-1.

■ The NiCd batteries provide the power for the production of x-rays. When the batteries lose their charge, they must be recharged using the standard wall power outlet. The batteries produce a low-voltage DC charge.

■ The DC chopper produces a pulsed DC that goes to the primary coil of the high-voltage transformer.

■ The high-voltage transformer produces the kilovoltage required to operate the x-ray tube. The output is high-voltage AC.

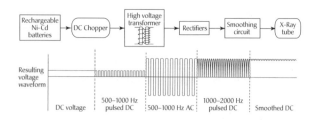

Figure 9-1 The major electrical components of a battery-powered portable x-ray machine. The associated voltage waveform is also shown. *(From Thompson MA, Hattaway MP, Hall JD, Dowd SB. Principles of imaging science and protection. Philadelphia: WB Saunders, 1994. Used with permission.)*

■ Rectifiers receive the high-voltage AC from the high-voltage transformer and convert it into a high-voltage pulsed DC with 100% ripple.

■ The smoothing circuit receives the pulsed DC from the rectifiers and performs a smoothing operation to reduce the ripple.

■ The voltage waveform (nearly constant) with reduced ripple is used to energize the x-ray tube to produce x-rays.

The battery-powered mobile x-ray unit ensures that the mA and kVp remain constant for the duration of the exposure. Additionally, the batteries provide power to all components of the machine, including the power to produce x-rays.

Mobile Units with High-Frequency Generators

Recently, mobile x-ray units with high-frequency generators have become popular for use in radiology. One of the significant advantages of the high-frequency generator is its compact design. In addition, the high-frequency generator (see Chapter 3) facilitates the use of less bulky transformers that can be placed within the x-ray tube housing (in some units).

■ The high-frequency generator converts the low-frequency AC (60 Hz) into high-frequency (kHz) pulsed DC, which is subsequently increased to kilovolts, rectified, and sent to the x-ray tube.

- The high-frequency generator produces a nearly constant voltage waveform with extremely low ripple ($< 1\%$).
- The high-frequency generator provides greater x-ray quantity and quality (effective energy). This factor makes the high-frequency generator significantly more efficient than the previous described generators. Higher exposure technique factors (mA and kVp), particularly with shorter exposure times, can be used to image critically ill patients, as well as large body regions, with optimal image quality.

High-frequency portable units are, to a certain extent, more costly, compared with the other two types of mobile units previously described.

Accessory Equipment

The accessory equipment for mobile radiographic systems should include grids, immobilizing devices, cassette holders, calipers, cloth (pillow case), a measuring tape, and a bottle of disinfectant.

Scattered Radiation Grids

Grids are described in Chapter 7. The purpose of a grid is to improve radiographic contrast by preventing scattered rays from reaching the film.

- Focused stationary grids with grid ratios of 6:1 or 8:1 are preferred over stationary, parallel-type grids.
- When using the grid, remember the relationships among the grid, the central ray of the x-ray beam, and the patient, to ensure optimal image quality.
- The grid must be used at its proper focal range.

Immobilizing Devices

To produce sharp images, patient immobilization is mandatory. The use of immobilization devices during portable radiography will assist in avoiding repeats resulting from patient motion.

- The use of an immobilizer should not delay the speed of the examination, however, particularly with patients who are critically ill.

■ Appropriate immobilizers for portable radiography include sandbags, masking tape, balsa wood, sheets, pads, and blocks of polyfoam.

Cassette Holders

Cassette holders are special metal frames intended to hold the cassette in place during the exposure.

■ Some cassette holders have a grid permanently mounted onto the holder frame.

■ These holders are especially useful for lateral and decubitus projections.

Calipers

Calipers are used to measure accurately the thickness of the anatomic region under investigation. The use of a caliper in portable radiography ensures that the correct exposure technique factors can be selected from the technique chart. This practice will always produce consistent results when patients have to be imaged on a daily basis.

Cloth Wrapper

A piece of cloth (sheet or pillowcase) should always be available to the technologist conducting a portable examination. Wrapping the cold cassette with a piece of cloth ensures patient comfort and keeps the cassette clean as well.

Disinfectant

All portable units should have the appropriate disinfectant to clean the cassette after use, especially when the cassette is contaminated with blood or body fluids.

Measuring Tape

A measuring tape should always be made available for portable radiography to ensure that the correct source-to-image receptor distance is used for the examination and to eliminate estimating the distance. Guessing the distance may result in the use of incorrect exposure technique factors and repeats from overexposures and underexposures.

FLUOROSCOPIC SYSTEMS

Mobile fluoroscopy has found applications in the operating room, gastrointestinal and vascular laboratories, emergency rooms, and orthopedic offices. Because technologists (in general) do not perform mobile fluoroscopy, only the basics are reviewed.

- Mobile fluoroscopy is usually performed by surgeons, radiologists, and by other physicians.
- Individuals who are not trained in the art and science of radiology should be trained in the principles and instrumentation aspects of fluoroscopy before they perform fluoroscopic examinations.

The major components of a mobile (portable) fluoroscopic imaging machine are the x-ray tube and generator, c-arm support, image intensifier tube, closed-circuit TV chain, control console, an image recording system, and automatic brightness control.

X-Ray Tube and Generator

The x-ray generator provides the necessary electrical power to the x-ray tube. Because these units must be lightweight and compact:

- High-frequency generators are used, which are efficient, small, and can be mounted on the unit itself.
  - These generators are generally rated at 1 to 4 kW of continuous power.
  - Tube currents and kVp generally range from 1 to 6 mA and 40 to 120 kVp, respectively, to accommodate the examination in the areas previously mentioned.
  - If the high-level fluoroscopic mode ("boost mode") is used, then the mA can approach 20.
  - Mobile fluoroscopic units can also be operated in the radiographic mode in conjunction with a grid and cassette that can be attached to the image intensifier tube. The x-ray generator must therefore be capable of providing higher mA values for radiography.
- The x-ray tube is usually a stationary-anode tube in most mobile fluoroscopic systems. These tubes have:

❑ Dual focal spots, a small focal spot (approximately 0.6 mm) for fluoroscopy, and a large focal spot (approximately 1.5 mm) for radiography.

❑ Collimators with copper beam-limiting filtration to reduce the dose to the patient and shape the beam to the area of interest.

❑ Fairly high heat storage capacities to accommodate lengthy fluoroscopic times.

C-Arm Support

The C-arm support describes a "C" with the x-ray tube mounted at one end and the image intensifier tube at the other end.

■ The C-arm allows for the patient to be positioned between the x-ray tube and image intensifier, which allows the operator free access to the patient.

■ The C-arm design also allows for a wide variety of movements, such as horizontal, vertical, panning, angled, and orbital movement to accommodate the requirements of various examinations.

Image Intensifier

The image intensifiers used in mobile systems are generally small. Six-inch input phosphor diameters are common.

■ Intensifiers can operate in several dual nodes, such as 9- and 6-inch, and 7- and 4-inch. Triple modes are also possible, such as the 9-, 6-, and 4.5-inch. In the smaller modes, the image is magnified and the radiation dose increases (see Chapter 8).

■ Larger intensifiers that have a 12-inch input phosphor diameter are also available, especially for use in vascular imaging during which a large field-of-view is necessary.

Closed-Circuit TV Chain

The closed-circuit TV chain includes the charge-coupled device (CCD) camera (TV camera tubes are not used in state-of-the-art units), coaxial cable, TV control electronics, and a TV monitor. (These components are described in Chapter 8.) However, the following points are noteworthy:

■ The CCD camera is coupled with the image intensifier and receives the light from the output phosphor.

- The CCD matrix array varies; however, 512 × 512 arrays are common.
- The CCD sends the output video signal via the coaxial cable to the TV electronics box for signal amplification and is subsequently sent to the TV monitor.

TV Monitor

The TV monitor uses the signal from the CCD camera to display images for viewing.

- In general, most systems use two monitors: one to display the current image and the other to display a previously acquired image.
- Images can be displayed in any orientation to facilitate diagnosis via a keyboard.

Control Console

The control console allows the operator to communicate with the system.

- The console displays all exposure parameters (kVp, mA, fluoroscopy time).
- Separate controls are also available for radiography.

Image Recording

There are essentially two approaches to recording the fluoroscopic image. These include radiography and multi-format camera recording.

- To record hard copy images by means of radiography, a cassette holder and a grid can be attached to the image intensifier tube. Radiography exposure technique factors are used to record these images.
- Multi-format cameras can also be used to record images on film.

Automatic Brightness Control

Mobile fluoroscopic imaging units are provided with automatic brightness control (ABC) systems to adjust the mA and kVp simultaneously as the thickness of the object being examined varies.

- ABC systems ensure uniform picture brightness on the TV monitor as the part thickness changes. This system

is important so as not to change the contrast percepti-
bility of the observer.
- ABC systems also provide a method of keeping the dose
  to the patient at minimal levels during operation of the
  unit.

Digital Image Capture

Most mobile fluoroscopic imaging systems can operate in the
digital imaging mode. Essential features include:

- Digitizing the output video signal from the CCD camera.
- Digital subtraction angiography mode (see Chapter 8),
  as well as nonsubtracted digital angiography mode are
  possible with varying frame rates (Gingold, 1996).
- Image acquisition matrix of $512 \times 512 \times 8$ bit to 10 bit
  depth ensures a wide dynamic range.
- Image storage on magnetic disks or laser optical disks.
- A variety of image processing operations, such as filter-
  ing for edge enhancement and noise reduction.
- A paper printer to provide a hard copy of digital images.
- A networking system to facilitate communication of
  images, such as sending them (images) to a picture
  archiving and communication system (PACS). PACS can
  provide the capability to also send images to laser print-
  ers in the department (Gingold, 1996).

MINI C-ARM FLUOROSCOPIC SYSTEMS

Recently, mini C-arm mobile fluoroscopic imaging systems
have been introduced and dedicated for imaging extremities
(Schueler, 2000).

- Major components of a mini C-arm system consist of a
  mini C-arm that supports a low-powered x-ray tube and
  an intensifier, a CCD camera, an integrated keyboard,
  floppy disk storage units, and a thermal printer for hard
  copying.
- The distance from the x-ray tube to the image intensifier is approximately 14 to 15 inches.
- The field-of-view (FOV) varies from 7 cm to 13 cm.
- The x-ray tube is a stationary-anode tube with extremely small focal spot sizes (0.1 to 0.3 mm). Low-powered

    generators allow operation at 40 to 70 kVp and 25 to
    150 mA.

■ Some units use a micro-channel plate intensifier; cesium
    iodide image intensifiers are used in others.

■ Digital image acquisition and processing are also avail-
    able on these units.

■ "Because these systems operate at low power, exposure
    rates are relatively low at normal source-to-skin distance
    (less than 0 • 5R/min [0.129 mC/kg • min] at 3 cm from
    the from the image intensifier). If geometric magnifica-
    tion is used to show finer detail, the skin exposure rate
    will naturally increase" (Gingold, 1996).

Portable radiography and fluoroscopy require a good deal
of understanding of the equipment components and principles
of operation. These criteria provide the expertise necessary to
ensure not only the best possible image quality, but also the
speed and accuracy required when imaging patients who are
critically ill or traumatized, as well as patients having surgical
procedures.

CHAPTER 10

Equipment Maintenance: Continuous Quality Improvement

Chapter at a glance

The optimization of patient care, image quality, radiation protection of patients and personnel, and cost control in the radiography department depends on the effectiveness of a *continuous quality improvement* (CQI) program.

In 1991 the Joint Commission on the Accreditation of Healthcare Organization (JCAHO) introduced the CQI concept to address a wide scope of issues relating to *quality assurance* (QA) and *quality control* (QC), older concepts designed to ensure optimal performance of personnel and equipment in the care and management of the patient in radiology.

This chapter examines the fundamental principles of QC rather than QA and CQI, since the principal activities of technologists are related to the performance and the on-going evaluation of the equipment used to image patients. Specifically highlighted are the basic tools for QC testing and the parameters for QC monitoring, the basic QC tests and tolerance units for radiography and fluoroscopy and for film processors, as well as repeat-reject film analysis.

DEFINITIONS

CQI programs are based on the use of QA and QC. Therefore it is essential that the technologist have a clear understanding of the meaning of these terms to assume the proper responsibility in the department.

Quality Control

The National Council on Radiation Protection and Measurements (NCRP) defines QC as the following:

> "Quality control is a series of distinct technical procedures which ensure the production of a satisfactory product. Its aim is to provide quality that is not only satisfactory and diagnostic, but also dependable and economic."

An effective QC program includes the following three steps:

- *Acceptance testing.* This represents the first step of a QC program and should be conducted by a medical physicist or a biomedical engineer. Acceptance testing is performed to ensure that new imaging and film processing equipment meet the manufacturer's stated performance specifications.

- *Routine performance evaluation.* This step is conducted by technologists, as well as medical physicists (who perform the more invasive and complex testing of the equipment). Various equipment parameters are tested and the results are evaluated. If the results fall within defined tolerance limits or acceptance criteria, then the equipment passes the test. If tolerance limits are not met, then corrective action must be taken. QC tests must be conducted in a systematic manner to ensure accurate results.

■ *Corrective action.* This step involves servicing and repairing the equipment so as to perform within acceptable limits. This step is important to maintain image quality standards while keeping the radiation dose as low as is reasonably achievable.

Quality Assurance

As noted by the NCRP, QA is a "comprehensive concept" and it is:

> "...an all-encompassing program, including quality control, that extends to administrative, educational, and preventive maintenance methods. It includes a continuing evaluation of the adequacy and effectiveness of the overall imaging program, with a view to initiating corrective measures when necessary."

■ Although QC deals with equipment monitoring and the technical aspects of performance and maintenance, QA deals specifically with management and administrative practices that optimize patient throughput and safety and ensures prompt interpretation of the patient's films (images).

■ QA also addresses the costs and benefits associated with the program, for example, costs that are related to personnel, test equipment, and a decrease in patient throughput as a result of testing, must be considered.

■ The implementation and continued operation of an effective QA program rest with radiologists and management personnel.

Continuous Quality Improvement

Although QA-QC programs play a significant role in ensuring image quality standards and optimizing patient care and image interpretation time, they have limitations. As noted by Papp:

> "It was segmented in approach, because each department in a facility monitored and evaluated their own structural outcomes, creating a tendency to view individual performances rather than the process or system in which that individual was functioning. In turn, the program was externally motivated, because

its emphasis was on demonstrating compliance with externally developed standards. As long as the standards were met, no further work was required to improve the system" (1998).

In 1991 the JCAHO introduced the notion of CQI as a means of overcoming the limitations of QA-QC programs and to raise the level of involvement of all employees in ensuring a quality product from the facility.

- Other terms synonymous with CQI are *total quality management* (TQM), *total quality improvement* (TQI), *total quality control* (TQC), *total quality leadership* (TQL), and *statistical quality control* (SQC).
- CQI is an on-going activity based on W. Edwards Deming's (a professor of business statistics) philosophy that he used to further Japan's industrial recovery after World War II. *Deming's philosophy* includes 14 points to help organizations develop CQI programs.

It is not within the scope of this text to describe Deming's 14 points. The main focus here is to highlight the essential elements of quality control, rather than continuous quality improvement.

Format of a QC Test

There are several formats used to guide the technologist-medical physicist in conducting QC tests, all of which include some common elements.

A typical format for conducting a QC test is as follows:

- *Aim.* Statement of the purpose of the test.
- *Equipment needed.* List of all the equipment required to conduct the test.
- *Procedure.* List of steps on how to use the equipment to conduct the test.
- *Results.* Record of the data (numerical, image, or graphical display) obtained after all procedural steps have been conducted.
- *Discussion.* Description or discussion of the results obtained, including a statement of the tolerance limits or acceptance criteria for the parameter tested, and whether the tolerance limits have been met. (Test procedure limitations should be recorded as well.)

- ■ *Action.* Statement of whether the equipment has passed the test or whether corrective action is required. (Frequency of testing for the particular parameter should be recorded as well.)

A record of all tests conducted should be kept in a manual for accreditation purposes and to provide data on the history of testing so as to detect trends in the performance of the equipment.

TOOLS FOR QC TESTING

There is a variety of tools available for QC testing, ranging from simple to complex, depending on the level of testing.

Levels of QC Testing

Three levels of QC testing have been identified in the literature. They are:

- ■ *Level I.* These tests are simple, noninvasive, and require the expertise of any technologists with basic radiography training to perform them. Examples include screen-film contact test, collimation test using 8-pennies, and the spinning top test for checking the accuracy of the exposure timer of single-phase generator units.
- ■ *Level II.* These tests are noninvasive, complex, and require the expertise of a technologist who has had additional technical training in QC procedures. These tests use tools that are considered more advanced and require careful handling and placement during the QC test procedure. Examples of these tests include kVp accuracy test, timing and mA linearity test, and half-value layer (HVL) test for beam quality assessment.
- ■ *Level III.* These tests are considered invasive, complex, and require the expertise of the medical physicist and/or biomedical engineer. Examples of these tests include timer and kVp accuracy testing using oscilloscopes and other equipment coupled with the x-ray tube and high-voltage generator. Additionally, medical physicists in general conduct dose assessment tests. This level of testing may also involve some degree of collaboration between the medical physicist-engineer and the QC technologist.

This chapter addresses Level I and Level II QC testing only.

Basic Test Tools

The QC test tools reported here are common tools that are used for Level I and Level II testing. It is not within the scope of this section to describe all the tools available. However, basic tools for radiographic fluoroscopic and processor QC are highlighted.

- **Sensitometer.** This tool is used in the radiology darkroom to produce an accurately reproducible light exposure on a film. When this film is processed in the film processor, the result is a *sensitometry* strip that contains a range of density steps.

- **Densitometer.** This device measures the optical density in any region of a film. For example, the optical densities of the sensitometry strip can be measured by the densitometer and the values plotted as a function of the log relative exposure values to produce a film *characteristic curve.*

- **Step wedge or penetrometer.** This wedge is made of aluminum with a range of steps varying from approximately 11 to 21. This wedge can be used in a number of QC tests such as identifying problems involving processor or radiographic exposure.

- **Thermometer.** This tool is used to check the temperatures of film processing solutions such as the developer and fixer.

- **Perforated metal mesh.** This mesh is used to examine film-screen contact. Poor contact will result in density variations on the film and blurring that can lead to diagnostic interpretation errors.

- **Collimator test tools.** "Homemade" and commercial tools are included, which check the alignment of the collimator light field with that of the radiation field shaped by the collimator. Homemade tools include 8-pennies, as well as metal washers and paper clips. One commercially available tool is a flat plate with a rectangular pattern (14 × 18 cm) etched onto the surface. Radiographic and fluoroscopic collimation accuracy can be checked using this tool.

- **Beam alignment tool.** This QC test tool is a plastic tube containing two steel balls (1.6 mm in diameter), placed precisely over each other and separated by a distance of approximately 15.2 cm. The tool provides a simple pass-fail test to indicate whether the central ray of the x-ray beam is perpendicular to the image receptor, in non-angled beam procedures.

■ *Spinning top.* This is a metal disk containing a hole on the periphery of the disks, on which sits on a central spindle that allows the disk to rotate. The top is used to check the accuracy of the exposure timer of single-phase x-ray machines.

■ *Synchronous spinning top.* This spinning top plugs into the AC wall outlet and is used to test the accuracy of exposure timers for three-phase generator units.

■ *kVp test tools.* There are several tools for checking the kVp accuracy, such as the Wisconsin cassette and the more recent test tools, such as ion chambers and photo diodes, as well as the oscilloscope.

■ *Focal spot test tools.* There are several tools available to measure the size of the focal spot of an x-ray tube. These include the pinhole and slit cameras, star test patterns, and bar patterns.

■ *Tomographic test tools.* These tools include a set of plastic disks to measure parameters such as section thickness and level and uniformity of exposure.

■ *Fluoroscopic QC test tools.* A wide range of test tools are available and are intended for Level III testing conducted by the medical physicist-biomedical engineer. One common test tool, however, is the resolution test tool, which is a wire mesh specifically intended to check the resolution as seen on the fluoroscopic television monitor.

PARAMETERS FOR QC MONITORING

There are at least five key components that require QC monitoring in a radiology department. These are:

■ *Basic characteristics of the x-ray imaging system.* For radiographic systems, a QC program should include routine evaluation of filtration, collimation, focal spot size, kVp and timer accuracy, mA linearity, and exposure reproducibility. For fluoroscopy, basic QC tests include the entrance skin exposure rate, automatic exposure control systems, and the resolution as seen on the television monitor. For conventional tomography (which is becoming less common in modern imaging departments), the section thickness and level, as well as the exposure uniformity, should be evaluated.

- **Protective aprons and gloves.** Protective garments must be checked for any defects such as tears, holes, and cracks.

- **Cassettes and grids.** Cassette parameters include film-screen contact, screen condition, light leaks, and artifact identification; grid parameters include alignment, focal distance, and artifact identification.

- **Darkroom and film processors.** Although there are several elements to be evaluated, major parameters include light and leakage testing, processor cleaning and maintenance, and processor monitoring to include sensitometry and densitometry.

- **View boxes or film illuminators.** The parameters to be evaluated for view boxes are the consistency of light output (or viewbox illumination) using photometric analysis, as well as viewbox surface conditions.

ACCEPTANCE CRITERIA–TOLERANCE LIMITS

The results of all QC testing must be carefully evaluated by the technologist and medical physicist, and a decision must be made to determine whether the results are acceptable or not acceptable. In arriving at a decision, it is beneficial to establish acceptance criteria or tolerance limits, certain defined limits that have ± values.

- *Tolerance limits* can be expressed quantitatively, such as ± 0.5 or ± 3% or ≤ 1.3 mC per kg per min. These are objective standards.

- Tolerance limits can also be expressed qualitatively, such as pass-fail, or no significant areas of poor contact seen. These are subjective standards and they are based on the opinions of QC personnel, including radiologists.

- If the results of a QC test fall within the tolerance limit, then the test results are considered acceptable. If the results exceed the tolerance limits, then the test indicates that the equipment performance is unacceptable.

Tolerance limits for selected QC tests are provided in the next session.

CONTROL CHARTS

QC testing involves recording all measurements taken during the evaluation of the equipment. To record these measurements, control charts are essential in a QC program, particularly in a processor QC program.

- A *control chart* or *trend chart* as it is frequently called, shows a graphic illustration of the performance of the equipment or the parameter measured as a function of time.

- A control chart allows for an easy assessment of the data compared with analyzing numbers recorded in table form.

- Usually a control chart consists of an average (or mean) baseline performance level and upper and lower control limits. If the equipment operating levels fall outside these limits, then corrective action must be taken. If the operating levels approach the upper or lower control limits but do not exceed them, then this is an indication of the beginning of a problem that will need to be addressed. In this case, the control chart will show a trend or drift.

BASIC QC TESTS FOR RADIOGRAPHY

QC tests for radiography can range from simple tests that can be conducted by technologists to complex tests that require the expertise of a QC technologist-medical physicist, specifically trained in advanced QC testing and evaluation.

In this section, only basic QC tests are reviewed. The review is not described in any detail how to conduct the test (procedures), but it focuses on the purpose of the test, the frequency of testing, and the tolerance limits or acceptance criteria. Technologists must refer to textbooks and lecture notes for details on how the test should be conducted.

Major Parameters and Tolerance Limits

The NCRP and other organizations such as the American College of Medical Physicists (ACMP) and the American Association of Physicists in Medicine (AAPM) have indicated that basic tests for radiographic QC include x-ray tubes and collimators, x-ray generators, grids, film cassette, in addition to a visual inspection of the equipment.

■ *Visual inspection*
   ❏ The purpose of visual inspection is to examine all aspects of the equipment to ensure that they will provide for comfort and safety of both patients and personnel during the examination.
   ❏ Some items are inspected on a daily basis; others will require annual inspection.
   ❏ The tolerance limits are qualitative. All problems and potential problems must be reported to the manager and clinical engineer-medical physicist who should address the means to rectify problems that pose a danger to patients and personnel.
■ *Filtration*
   ❏ The purpose of filtration is to protect the patient by removal of the low-energy x-rays from the beam. Since inherent filtration cannot be measured, the HVL of the beam must be measured. The HVL is that thickness of aluminum required to reduce the beam intensity to one half of its original value. "It is not a measure of the amount of aluminum in the beam" (NCRP, 1988).
   ❏ The frequency of filtration (HVL) checks is annually.
   ❏ The tolerance limit for filtration depends on the kVp used. The minimum HVL in millimeters of aluminum for the following kVp is:
      50 kVp: 1.2 mm aluminum
      70 kVp: 1.5 mm aluminum
      90 kVp: 2.5 mm aluminum
■ *Collimation*
   ❏ The purpose of the collimation QC test is to check the alignment of the light field of the field of the collimator and the radiation field shaped by the collimator. These two fields must be in perfect alignment. Automatic collimation (positive beam limitation, PBL) should also be tested to ensure that the x-ray field size is not larger than the size of the image receptor.
   ❏ The tolerance limit for light field and x-ray field alignment is such that the misalignment must not be greater than ±2% of the source-to-image receptor distance (SID). For PBL systems the misalignment must not be greater than ± 3% of the SID.

- *Focal spot size.* The size of the focal spot affects the detail of the image.
  - ❏ The purpose of QC test for focal spot size is to ensure that the size of the focal spot is within acceptable limits.
  - ❏ QC test should be performed only during the acceptance testing stage, or it can be checked annually as well.
  - ❏ The measured size may be 50% greater than the stated size and still be within acceptable limits. Therefore for a 0.3 mm focal spot size, 0.45 can be tolerated. If the size is greater, then the x-ray tube should be changed.
- *kVp accuracy.* The kVp affects both the dose the patient receives and the image contrast. Low kVp means greater contrast but higher patient dose resulting from the predominance of the photoelectric absorption.
  - ❏ The purpose of the kVp QC test is to check the accuracy of the kVp. The technologist wants to find out whether the measured kVp is the same as the setting on the control panel.
  - ❏ Test should be performed annually.
  - ❏ Tolerance limit for the kVp accuracy test is ± 5% of the value set on the control panel. For example, if 80 kVp is set up for the examination, ± 4 kVp is acceptable for the measured value (76 or 84 kVp would be acceptable). As noted by Bushong (2001), although a 2 to 3 kVp variation will "measurably affect patient dose and image optical density," a 4 to 5 kVp difference will influence image contrast.
- *Exposure timer accuracy.* The exposure time affects image density and dose through a direct proportionality. If the exposure time is doubled, then the dose and optical density are increased by a factor of two.
  - ❏ The technologist can set exposure timers manually or they can be used in the automatic mode of operation.
  - ❏ The purpose of the QC test for exposure timing using the timer in the manual mode is to ensure that the measured time is the same as that set on the control panel. The purpose of the test for the automatic timer is to check that the exposure stops after the correct film density has been detected.

❑ Exposure timers should be checked annually.
❑ The tolerance limits are as follows:
❑ For manual timers:
  ● Accuracy should be within ±5% of the time set on the unit for times greater than 10 milliseconds (ms).
  ● For exposure times of 10 ms or less, an accuracy of ±20% is acceptable.
❑ For automatic timers:
  ● For all objects of varying thicknesses imaged, the densities of all films should be within ±0.10 of each other. All films should have the same density for proper functioning automatic exposure timers.

■ *Exposure linearity.* The same mAs values for different combinations of mA and time settings that produce the same exposure output is referred to as the exposure linearity.
  ❑ Purpose of the exposure linearity QC test is to check that the same exposure output is measured for different combinations of mA and time that produce the same mAs.
  ❑ This test should be done once a year.
  ❑ The tolerance limit for this test is that the linearity should be less than or equal to ±10%.

■ *Exposure reproducibility.* When the same mA, time, and kVp values are used repeatedly, the exposure output for each exposure should be the same.
  ❑ This test should be done annually.
  ❑ The tolerance limit is that the output exposure should not vary by more than ±5%.

■ *Film-screen contact*
  ❑ The purpose of this QC test is to ensure that cassettes provide the best possible contact between the screen and the film.
  ❑ This test should be performed one or two times a year.
  ❑ The tolerance limits are as follows:
    ● Blurred areas at the edges of the film may be acceptable.
    ● Blurred areas in the middle of the film are not acceptable and corrective action should be taken.

- ■ *Viewbox illumination*
  - ❑ The purpose of the QC test for film illuminators is to ensure that the brightness level of the viewbox is consistent.
  - ❑ This test should be performed annually.
  - ❑ The tolerance limit is that the brightness level should not vary by more than ±10% of the standard intensity.

Basic QC Tests for Conventional Tomography

Major Parameters and Tolerance Limits
Several parameters require QC monitoring. However, because conventional tomographic systems are becoming obsolete, only two parameters—section level and section thickness—are highlighted.

- ■ *Section level and thickness*
  - ❑ The purpose of the QC test for section level and section thickness is to ensure that they are accurate and that optimal image detail is obtained.
  - ❑ Testing frequency varies depending on the problems encountered.
  - ❑ The tolerance limit for the section level should be within ±5 mm of the setting. For section thickness, Gray, et al. (1983) point out:

    On linear systems, there should be a zone of sharp focus with a visible, although blurred, region on both sides. The thickness of the region in focus may be approximated by measuring the width of the mesh that is in focus and dividing by two. The section thickness depends on the amplitude (tomographic angle). For example, the section thickness at 40, 30, and 10 degrees is 1.4 mm, 2.0 mm, and 6.0 mm, respectively.

Basic QC Tests for Fluoroscopic Systems

There are three main system components of a fluoroscopic imaging unit that should be monitored by QC testing. These components include the x-ray tube and generator, the image intensifier tube, and the closed-circuit x-ray television system.

The parameters for QC testing are numerous, including filtration, focal spot size, kVp accuracy, mA linearity, exposure reproducibility, grid uniformity and alignment, automatic brightness control, maximum exposure rates, resolution (spatial and contrast), and the television monitor performance.

Major Parameters and Tolerance Limits

It is not within the scope of this chapter to describe all the fluoroscopic parameters that require QC monitoring. However, a few are highlighted. The medical physicist or the QC technologist conducts most of the QC tests for fluoroscopy.

- *Maximum fluoroscopic exposure rate*
  - ❑ The purpose of testing the exposure rate is to ensure that the fluoroscopic system provides an exposure rate that will image patients of all sizes, with optimal image quality.
  - ❑ The test should be conducted semiannually.
  - ❑ The tolerance limit for this test indicates the entrance skin exposure rate should not exceed 2.6 mC/kg/min (10 R/min) or 100 mGy/min(10 R/min).
- *Television monitor resolution*
  - ❑ This test uses a copper mesh test pattern consisting of eight pie-shaped segments having 16, 20, 24, 30, 35, 40, 50, and 60 holes per inch.
  - ❑ The purpose of this test is to evaluate the resolution capability of the fluoroscopic imaging system as displayed on the television (TV) monitor.
  - ❑ The test should be performed annually.
  - ❑ The tolerance limits for this test indicate that for a 23 cm (9-inch) image intensifier tube coupled to a standard TV display system, the minimum mesh holes per inch visualized should be 20 to 24 in the center of the display and 20 at the edge of the display (Gray, et al., 1983).
- *Visual inspection.* Technologists should perform a visual inspection at least every 6 months of a wide range of equipment components to ensure not only optimal system performance, but also patient and personnel safety and comfort during the procedure. Examples of components requiring visual inspection include the fluoroscopic tower and table locks, protective curtain and aprons,

Bucky slot cover, exposure switch, compression device, table angulation and motion, fluoroscopic cumulative timer, and collimator shutters.

QC FOR X-RAY FILM PROCESSORS

Film processing requires at least two elements: a darkroom and a film processor.

Darkroom and Safelight Testing

The darkroom is an integral area in the radiology department for several reasons:

- It provides storage area for films and chemical solutions.
- It protects unexposed films from light and radiation fog.
- It provides a controlled environment for handling processing chemicals—acetic acid, glutaraldehyde, phenol, hydroquinone—and is well ventilated so as to control chemical fumes and vapors.

An essential specification of the darkroom is the safelight—a source of light that provides proper illumination to allow the technologists to handle both exposed and unexposed films without fogging them. As noted by Papp, a film "should be able to remain in safelighting for at least 40 seconds without becoming fogged. Safelights should be mounted at least 3 to 4 feet from feed trays or loading counters" (1998). The type of safelight depends on the type of films used in the department.

- For blue violet–sensitive film, an amber safe light with a Kodak Wratten 6B filter (amber plastic/glass) or a Kodak Mor-Light is used.
- For orthochromatic film, a red safelight filter, such as Kodak's GBX, is used.

An important QC test is Safelight Testing. In this test, it is mandatory to use a densitometer to measure the optical density of the films tested.

- The purpose of this test is to check that the safelight will not fog the film for the duration of the time it is handled in the darkroom.
- This test should be done semiannually.

- The tolerance limits for this test, as noted by the NCRP, are:

  "Exposure of test film for one minute in the darkroom with safelight on should produce less than a 0.05 increase in the mid-density portion of the film (i.e., a density of about 1.20). Ideally, less than a 0.05 increase should be obtained with the two minute exposure to the darkroom lights" (1990).

Processor QC: Components

Several authors (Bushong, 2001; Gray, 1997; Papp, 1998) have identified at least four major components of an effective processor QC program. These components include chemical activity, processor cleaning, processor maintenance, and processor monitoring.

- *Processor chemical activity.* This activity refers to the integrity of the processing solutions. Variables such as the temperature of the solution, processing time, replenishment rate, the pH of the solution, and the specific gravity, all affect the chemical activity.
  - ❑ Developer solution temperature should not vary by more than ±0.5° F (0.3° C) from the manufacturer's specifications. Fixer and wash water temperature should be kept within ±5° F (3° C).
  - ❑ The processing time for the developer should be ±2% to 3% of the manufacturer's specifications.
  - ❑ The replenishment rate should be within ±5% of the manufacturer's specification.
  - ❑ The pH of solutions should be within 10 and 11.5. The pH plays a role in contrast and density of the film. Low pH values decrease film contrast and density.
  - ❑ The specific gravity for the developer and fixer should be within 1.07 to 1.10 and 1.077 to 1.110 with a variation of not more than ±0.004 from the manufacturer's specifications, respectively (Papp, 1998).
- *Processor cleaning.* Processor cleaning includes daily cleaning of the cross-over racks and weekly cleaning of the complete rack mechanism, as well as all processing tanks. Cleaning optimizes film processing and minimizes processing artifacts.
- *Processor maintenance.* Weekly observation of all mechanized parts and sufficient lubrication ensures smooth movement of the film through the processor. Additionally,

a preventive maintenance program optimizes processor performance.

- ■ *Processor monitoring.* A vital aspect of a processor QC program, processor monitoring involves daily sensitometry measurement and is performed using a sensitometer to produce a step-wedge pattern on film in a controlled manner. The film is processed and a sensitometric strip is obtained. Fog speed and contrast measurements are subsequently recorded on a control chart so as to evaluate daily and monthly trends in the measurements.

Repeat Film Analysis

A *repeat film analysis* is an important part of a QC program. The central activity in a repeat film analysis is a careful and systematic assessment of the reasons why films have to be repeated or why they have been rejected.

- ■ The benefits of a repeat film analysis are to improve the efficiency of the examination, to reduce the costs associated with films and processing, and to minimize the dose to patients from repeat exposures.
- ■ The repeat film analysis includes collecting and sorting rejected films into various categories that identify the reasons films were discarded. Examples of these categories are poor positioning, poor density and contrast, blurring from patient motion, and the presence of artifacts and processing errors.

Finally, the repeat rate can be calculated knowing the total number of films used during the period of the study and the total number of patients involved.

- ■ For a repeat analysis to be valid, at least 250 patients are required (Bushong, 2001). Papp (1998) identifies two kinds of repeat rates: casual repeat rate and total repeat rate.
- ■ The percentage casual repeat rate is a ratio of the number of repeats from a specific cause to the total number of repeats multiplied by 100.
- ■ The percentage total repeat rate is a ratio of the number of repeat films to the total number of films produced multiplied by 100.

- The tolerance limits for a repeat film analysis are such that repeat rates should not be greater than 4% to 6% (Papp, 1998). The percentage repeat rate for each category should range from 2% to 5%. When repeat rates exceed these limits, corrective action is required.

RECORD KEEPING

It is mandatory that all QC testing be documented and that all records be kept in a manual. This is important not only for accreditation purposes, but also, and more importantly, to optimize the effectiveness and quality of the QC program and to observe trends in the history of the program.

BENEFITS OF A CQI PROGRAM

The overall benefits of a CQI program include:
- Optimization of image quality.
- Reduction of doses to both patients and personnel.
- Reduction of costs to the patient and the imaging facility.
- Motivation of personnel to produce the best possible image and take pride in their work.
- Active participation of all personnel in the learning process.

Index